A Matter of Life and Death:

Health, Illness and Medicine in McLean County, 1830-1995

by
Lucinda McC

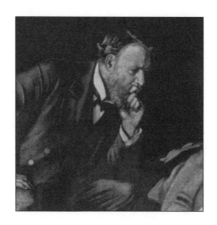

Library of Congress Cataloging-in-Publication Data

Beier, Lucinda McCray,
  A matter of life and death : health, illness and medicine in
McLean County, 1830-1995 / by Lucinda McCray Beier.
    p. cm.
  Includes bibliographical references and index.
  ISBN 0-943788-09-9
  1. Medicine--Illinois--McLean County--History. 2. Medical care--
Illinois--McLean County--History. 3. Public health--Illinois--McLean
County--History. I. Title.
  [DNLM: 1. History of Medicine, 19th Cent.--Illinois. 2. History
of Medicine, 20th Cent.--Illinois. 3. Delivery of Health Care--history--
Illinois. 4. Public Health--history--Illinois. 5. Health Personnel--
history--Illinois. WZ 70 AI3 B4m 1996]
R210.M35B45 1996
610'.9773'59--dc20
DNLM/DLC   96-29270
for Library of Congress   CIP

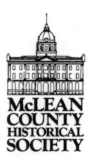

**McLEAN
COUNTY
HISTORICAL
SOCIETY**

Published by The McLean County Historical Society
Copyright © 1996, Lucinda McCray Beier
Cover and book design, Conley Art Studio
Printed by Bloomington Offset Process, Inc.

This publication is made possible in part by a grant from the
Illinois Humanities Council, the National Endowment for the
Humanities, and the Illinois General Assembly.

For my father, Dr. Robert Myles McCray,
the best healer I know.

Contents

Acknowledgments

No book is truly written alone. However, few books have benefited as much from collective effort and commitment as this one. For their enthusiasm and hard work, I wish to thank the community volunteers who explored McLean County's history of health, illness and medicine with me: Margaret Esposito, John Krueger, Nadine Reining, Madge Williams, Deborah Finfgeld, Christine Kibler, Michael Robak, Corlin Ferguson, and Ruth Carpenter. I also want to thank the oral history interviewees who donated their time to this project.

I am very grateful to staff members at the Old Courthouse Museum in Bloomington, Illinois, including Preston Hawks, Michelle McNabb and Patty Wagner, for the time and effort they devoted to this project. In particular, I want to thank Susan Hartzold, the museum's curator, who supported project research at every turn and made it possible for the arguments made in this book to be visualized in a temporary museum exhibit. I also want to thank Greg Koos, museum director, visionary and optimist, for asking me to do this project and steadfastly believing it would be completed.

Many thanks to Professor Norman Gevitz, Director of the Medical Humanities Department at the University of Illinois, Chicago, for reading several early chapters of the book manuscript. His comments were both useful and encouraging. I am also grateful to Kathleen and Loy Conley for their expert and patient editing which made the manuscript a book.

I gratefully acknowledge the financial support provided by the Illinois Humanities Council. I also wish to thank Julie Payne, of BroMenn Healthcare and Pam Meiner, of St. Joseph Medical Center, for both the personal contributions and the organizational resources they brought to the project. Thanks are also due to the McLean County Health Department, Mennonite College of Nursing, Illinois Wesleyan University's College of Nursing, the McLean County Medical Society and the Sisters of the Third Order of St. Francis for providing access to their records. Many thanks to the Bloomington-Normal Black History Project and Cynthia Baer for sharing their oral history transcripts with me. I am also grateful to my employer, the College of Arts and Sciences of Illinois State University, for supporting my participation in this project.

I want to thank Dr. Elizabeth Roberts, Director of the Center for North-West Regional Studies at Lancaster University (Great Britain), for introducing me to the practice of oral history.

Elizabeth's expertise, scholarship, encouragement and friendship fostered my interest in twentieth-century social history and gave me a powerful new method for exploring it.

Finally, I must thank my family. During the past year, when this book truly became a matter of life and death for me, consuming every evening and weekend, my husband, Lee, and sons, Joe, Jesse, Zach and Jake cheered my efforts and helped me to believe that the work was worth doing.

Introduction

In the beginning, there was the land — black, deep and rich — stoneless dirt that made hardscrabble farmers from New England and Lancashire figure they'd died and gone to heaven. There were clear streams, towering hardwoods, coal deposits and game animals to nurture settlement. There were also unforgiving winters, murderous summers, vicious mosquitoes and a host of diseases to challenge the migrants of European and African heritage who in the early nineteenth century came to what would later be called McLean County, Illinois.[1]

Those migrants came laden with the supplies and tools they knew were necessary to set up housekeeping in an "unimproved" (and unspoiled) natural environment. They also carried with them the cultural baggage of nineteenth-century Western civilization. They brought Bibles, pianos, guns, dress patterns and recipes. They also brought contemporary ideas about health, illness and healing; bottles filled with medical ingredients; surgical instruments; and books of instructions which became guides to survival for pioneer households — matters of life and death.

Birth, illness and dying are universal human experiences. However, each physical environment produces its own variations on these common themes, and each society develops its own particular ways of meeting these shifting challenges. This book traces the ways residents of McLean County have dealt with childbearing, infant care, illness, injury, handicap, old age, and dying, from the early days of settlement (*circa* 1830); through the late nineteenth-century development of a professional medical establishment; through the early twentieth-century expansion of public health and medical services; through the period of miracle medicine and surgery following World War II; to the era of reexamination and reorganization of health services in the late twentieth century. It considers the experiences of sufferers and healers, practitioners and patients. In considering changing expectations of health and medical care, it observes fundamental shifts in our

1

world view and in our perception of the elements necessary to support an acceptable quality of life. It also argues that McLean County exemplifies, in microcosm, the development of the modern American health care delivery system.

History is all about change and continuity. Theories and practices regarding health and medical care have, perhaps, changed more rapidly and radically than any other part of our culture. Nowadays, it would be unthinkable to treat a fractured limb without an x-ray; yet, one hundred years ago (Roentgen first identified x-rays in 1895) it would have been unimaginable to use for this purpose something which so smacked of magic and quackery. Nowadays, we assume that most illnesses are caused by the microscopic organisms we call germs; 140 years ago, when Pasteur was just beginning to be concerned about the diseases of wine and beer, elite physicians debated whether "miasmas" or contagion caused fevers and assumed that teething often killed infants. Yet, despite many changes, older ways of thinking about health and illness remain in living memory and influence our health practices. We still warn our children not to get their feet wet and put undershirts on babies in order to protect them from illness. We still smear camphorated ointments on our chests to relieve congestion. We still eat chicken soup, drink whiskey and call our mothers when we get sick. One era's official academic medicine becomes the next era's old wive's tales. Our collective memories are sturdy and conservative. Thus, we will begin this introductory overview of the history of health, illness and medical care in McLean County with a brief tour of the theory which dominated the general approach to prevention and healing in the nineteenth century — humoral theory.

Evil Humors and Heroic Remedies

Since classical times, Europeans believed that the human body was governed by the presence and balance of four essential humors, each with its own quality. The phlegmatic humor was cold and damp; the melancholic humor was cold and dry; the sanguine humor was hot and wet; the choleric humor was hot and dry. Health depended upon a balance of these humors within the body. Illness was caused by their imbalance — by the invasion of noxious external materials or an unhealthy build-up of a single humor within the body. Prevention of illness required maintenance of humoral equilibrium; cure of illness depended upon restoring that equilibrium. Each individual body was thought to have its own unique humoral composition and to suffer ill-health in ways unique to that composition. Few specific diseases were identified, and even these (smallpox, for example) could, like other fevers, fluxes or dropsies, change character, depending upon the individual they affected and the means that were taken against them. Virtually all therapies produced evacuation of some kind — purging, sweating, vomiting and bleeding were usual. Counter-irritants, such as blistering or cupping, were also widely used. The stronger the ailment suffered, the stronger the remedy needed.

Although early nineteenth-century European medical scientists developed new organ-centered theories of pathology which allowed for the identification and classification of specific disease entities, mainstream therapeutic techniques remained stubbornly humoral until at least the end of the century. Indeed, so extreme were the methods of evacuation used during this century that it has been dubbed the period of "heroic medicine", during which people swallowed gargantuan doses of purgatives and had themselves bled and blistered in their efforts to drive from their bodies accumulations of destructive material and restore the balance of health.[2]

People did not expect medicine-taking to make them feel good. Indeed, they expected medicines to taste foul and to make them feel terrible. They *did* expect remedies to work by producing some obvious effect (often laxative or emetic). They hoped that the application of heroic therapies would make them well, but they did not confidently expect this result. All accounts of nineteenth-century illnesses, whether written by physicians or lay-people, are imbued with a fatalism which accepted that once illness had attacked, it would run its natural course, either killing its victim outright or leaving him or her weakened but fortunate to be alive. Death was an expected visitor in every home, and was thought to be quite natural at certain times of life. Infants, child-bearing women and old people were considered so vulnerable that death certificates often record simply one of these circumstances as sufficient explanation of cause of death.

Since it was so difficult to cure nineteenth-century illnesses, people tried very hard to prevent them. They took tonics to purify their blood. They took purgatives to clean themselves out. They tried to avoid the drafts, damp, and cold which were thought to cause upper respiratory illness. They also knew that it was a good idea to avoid immoderate eating and drinking, which caused digestive problems. Physical exercise in the fresh air, combined with a diet rich in dairy products and meat, were thought to help

3

prevent tuberculosis. Maintenance of a healthy digestive system and avoidance of certain foods (such as fresh fruit) were though to protect people from cholera. Keeping out of the night air was believed to ward off malaria. Nonetheless, illness and death were expected, while prevention and cure were merely hoped for.

Nineteenth-Century Health Care Delivery in McLean County

Early migrants to the Illinois Territory brought with them a "do-it-yourself" attitude which extended beyond house-building, farming and commerce to health care. They carried with them prepared remedies such as calomel (a mercury derivative used for intestinal disorders and fevers), quinine (used for fevers), paregoric and laudanum (opium derivatives used to combat pain and make sufferers sleep). They gathered herbs and made home remedies according to traditional recipes. They willingly accepted care from amateur and professional healers, but did not expect access to these services. The real authorities in matters of childbearing, child rearing, nursing and general health were the mature women among them. A doctor's advice was sought, if at all, only during times of sickness.

Many physicians were among the area's early settlers.[3] Most of these had learned their skills through a combination of apprenticeship and academic coursework; few expected to be able to depend exclusively upon doctoring for their livelihoods. Many farmed. Most compounded and sold medicines. Some taught school, became businessmen or went into politics. The physician's work was hard and not particularly well paid. Indeed, physicians' fees were not much larger in 1890 than they had been in 1840.[4] While doctors were respected members of their communities, neither their incomes nor their social status were nearly as great as they became during the second half of the twentieth century.

Until the late nineteenth century, virtually all health care took place in the sufferer's home.[5] Physicians, surgeons, bonesetters, midwives and nurses routinely visited patients, taking with them everything needed for treatment. As the population grew and towns developed, drug stores and doctors' and dentists' offices were established; however, home care remained customary well into the twentieth century. Even after hospitals began to be built during the 1880s, these institutions were regarded as existing primarily for the use of the very poor or those elderly people having no one to look after them at home. Only with the parallel twentieth-century developments of medical technology related to everyday diagnosis and treatment and the increasing cultural authority of physicians did the location of care shift from the sufferer's home to a medical institution (i.e., a doctor's office or hospital).[6]

The development and evolution of health care delivery in McLean County reflects national trends. In the nineteenth century, allopathic physicians competed in a relatively open medical marketplace with many other kinds of practitioners (homeopaths, osteopaths, herbalists, eclectics and others) and a host of patent medicine manufacturers and retailers. Public health measures consisted primarily of efforts to construct sewer and public water systems in urban areas and impose home quarantine on sufferers from certain contagious diseases. During years when smallpox and cholera epidemics threatened, communities made special efforts to clean up public nuisances such as open sewers and garbage dumps. Otherwise, health and illness were private matters, left to the discretion of individuals.

With the flood of late nineteenth- and early twentieth-century identification of the microscopic organisms causing specific disorders, and vaccines and antitoxins which could prevent these diseases, public health activities gathered new momentum, both nationally and locally. Diagnostic laboratories, health education, the anti-tuberculosis movement and immunization campaigns focused both resources and public attention on disease prevention and eradication. Although McLean County did not have its own health department until 1945, public health activities were undertaken by a variety of organizations and individuals, including Bloomington's own health department, the Cooperative Extension Service, the Red Cross, public schools and, of course, medical practitioners. Both world views and manners changed as people recognized their power over the invisible enemies which pervaded their lives. Mothers learned to sterilize baby bottles, towns legislated against spitting on the street, children learned to make war on flies, and the world began to believe that by identifying the agents of infectious diseases, it had taken the first step in destroying them entirely.

Hospitals

The closing years of the nineteenth century gave rise to a period of energetic hospital building. Between 1880 and 1920, three major hospitals and a tuberculosis sanitarium opened their doors in Bloomington-Normal, while smaller McLean County communities also developed residential health care facilities.[7] Hospital expansion paralleled the development of antiseptic and aseptic surgery, health care technology, medical specialties and modern nursing. As it became difficult, both to transport all necessary equipment to the patient's home and to make of that home a germ-free environment, sufferers became accustomed to receiving hospital treatment for an expanding array of conditions. For example, while virtually all babies born in the county were delivered at home before 1920, first middle-class and urban, then rural and working-class couples began to opt for hospital deliveries after that date. Surgical operations frequently performed in nineteenth-century homes were almost always performed in hospitals by the mid-twentieth century. And, while early hospitals made almost no provision for treating children, pediatric wards were common and well used by about 1930. Hospitals expanded their services, adding x-ray departments, laboratories, maternity wards and emergency rooms to ever increasing numbers of beds. Hospital treatment became part of most people's experience and was increasingly viewed as a necessity.[8] While hospitals continued to treat charity patients, who were charged little or nothing for the care they received, payment for hospital services was expected from those who could afford to pay. Beginning in the interwar period, and proliferating after World War II, hospital insurance schemes became the usual way for people to protect themselves from rising costs of hospital care.[9]

Reliance upon hospital treatment was closely associated with acceptance of the germ theory and implementation of first antiseptic, then aseptic surgical techniques. Nineteenth-century hospitals had been dogged by high rates of infection, to the extent that conditions such as "hospital" gangrene and puerperal fever were generally assumed to be by-products of hospital environments. No wonder patients and physicians preferred home care whenever feasible. However, hospital-related infections were less common once Listerian procedures, including rigorous disinfection and sterilization of surfaces, instruments, linens and the hands of staff members, became routine. As hospitalization and surgery became safer, more ambitious surgical operations were attempted and all types of surgery were performed more often. While in the 1890s the McLean County Medical Society had discussed the pros and cons of the risky new operation for appendicitis, by the 1920s tonsillectomies were routinely done to prevent childhood illnesses and local surgeons performed goiter surgery on groups of patients

6

who suffered and recovered together.[10]   Surgeons and patients alike relied increasingly upon hospital facilities and routines to provide convenient and safe environments for both operations and convalescence.

With the expansion of the surgical repertoire, a trend in favor of specialization began. Many general practitioners opted, first informally, later increasingly by means of board certification, for specialized practices. For the gynecologists, orthopedic surgeons, radiologists, anesthesiologists and other specialists of the 1920s onwards, the hospital became a professional home in a way that it had never been for the typical family doctor of the nineteenth and early twentieth centuries. Hospitals and specialists had a symbiotic relationship: the expansion of hospitals provided specialists with facilities and staff support for their activities, while the proliferation of medical specialties created a need and a market for the large diversified hospitals of the mid-twentieth century.

Nursing

To support both expanding patient populations and medical staffs, hospitals took the lead in training nurses. All Bloomington hospitals opened nursing schools, and student nurses did much of the work involved in running those hospitals.[11] In the early days, nurse training was short and practical. Courses lasted for two years and involved more on-the-job training, active patient care and custodial work than classroom education. Once past a probationary period, student nurses, who paid no tuition, received small stipends to do everything from mopping the floor to making cotton swabs. Once nurses completed their training, they tended to work as private duty nurses, since few staff positions existed.

This situation changed after World War II, when nurse training became increasingly academic, and hospitals required increasingly specialized skills in nursing personnel. The trend in favor of nurses seeking bachelor's degrees became well established and strong links between nurse training programs and degree-granting colleges or universities were forged.[12] Hospitals employed increasing numbers of graduate nurses as student nurses became less available and less qualified for much patient care. Private duty nursing declined as intensive care facilities were organized. Following the pattern established by physicians, nurses increasingly specialized, opting to work as surgical, obstetrical, mental health, pediatric, or trauma nurses.

The Age of Miracles

World War II was a watershed in the history of medicine and surgery, serving as a dividing line between the relatively traditional health concerns of the pre-war period and expectations and a period of explosive biomedical progress which radically altered people's expectations of health, illness and medical care. In the mid-1940s, penicillin was introduced to the civilian population. The illnesses people most feared and were most likely to die of changed dramatically. Their expectations of professional medicine and surgery also altered. With antibiotics, previously murderous infections were rendered almost harmless. Killers like erysipelas, scarlet fever and rheumatic fever virtually disappeared. With the introduction of streptomycin in the late 1940s, tuberculosis sanitariums emptied. Post-operative surgical infection ceased to be a major concern. And physicians were the gatekeepers, governing access to these miraculous substances and receiving credit from a grateful public for the wonders they wrought. The authority, social status and incomes of doctors skyrocketed.

The post-war decades witnessed one miracle after another in medicine and surgery. Open heart, organ transplant and neurosurgery; drug therapies for mental illnesses; vaccines for polio; Space Age diagnostic technology — there seemed to be nothing that medical science could not do. The general public gave up its fatalism regarding illness and death and its skepticism regarding medical care. People eagerly relinquished responsibility for all health decisions and health care to professional medical practitioners. McLean County again followed national trends, developing a flourishing array of health care providers. Bloomington-Normal became a full service medical center for an area extending beyond the county borders. Business boomed.

In the last decade of the twentieth century, however, McLean County residents, like other Americans, have been forced to stand back and reexamine the approaches to health care they have chosen. While modern medical capabilities are enormous, their cost is apparently limitless. Because they are too expensive to use, hospitals must compete for patients. Rural areas can no longer attract and keep the family doctors they need because cities offer better support services and higher incomes. Physicians must share decision-making about patient care with insurance companies and health care administrators.

Meanwhile, even miracle medicine has been unable to beat

its old adversary — death. Today's killers are a stubborn crew. In the place of the infections so feared by our nineteenth-century forebears, we are hounded by a host of chronic disorders. Cancers, cardiovascular diseases, AIDS, Alzheimer's Disease — all mock our lust for immortality. Our expectations inflated by two generations of biomedical miracles, we demand that our healers fix whatever is broken, and sue them if they are unable to comply. We reject the notion of natural death, seeking eternal youth and beauty.

Human beings are adaptable. They are problem solvers. Like those nineteenth-century pioneers who built businesses and cities in the midwestern wilderness, we are in the process of using our tools and our minds to refashion our health care system to address our needs. The exercise of looking back over nearly two centuries of health, illness and medical care in McLean County may help us to identify what we value most highly in order to determine how the health care delivery system of the future should appear. In any case, it will show us how we got to this point.

How Do We Know?

The past is a foreign country. We assemble our versions of it — histories — on the basis of a patchwork of evidence. Traditional historians of medicine have relied upon certain kinds of documentary materials, including published medical texts, institutional records, and records kept by professional organizations. This history makes use of these types of records. Published and unpublished contemporary works and histories have been mined to illuminate past understanding and experience of health, illness and medical care in McLean County. Local hospitals and nursing schools have maintained excellent collections of administrative records, newspaper clippings, marketing materials and photographs which have been made available to this project.[13] The McLean County Medical Society has also been extremely supportive, providing access to its records. Extensive use has been made of the holdings of the McLean County Historical Society's Stevenson-Ives Library, which contains collections of correspondence, personal documents including diaries and physicians' day books, historical business directories, census data and newspaper files. The David Davis Mansion has generously provided access to documents regarding the experiences of Judge David Davis and his wife, Sarah Davis.

Documentary evidence can provide only part of the story,

however. The project also depends upon material objects to indicate what past experience was like. The medicine bottles, surgical instruments, baby bottles, syringes and outhouses of an era predating plastics, disposable items, and flush toilets speak both of universal human needs and the extent to which daily life has changed in a very short time.

In addition, 31 oral history interviews were recorded with nurses, physicians, dentists and lay people who shared their own experiences of health, illness, childbearing, death, and health care with project volunteers. Unlike voiceless documents and artifacts, these respondents could provide explanations for what they had to say. More than any other kind of historical source, they put a human face on past experience. This book owes the interview respondents an enormous debt of gratitude. They are its heart and soul.

1 Early Days: Suffering in McLean County

A peculiar stagnant smell hung over the anchorage — a smell of sodden leaves and rotting tree trunks. I observed the doctor sniffing and sniffing, like someone tasting a bad egg.

"I don't know about treasure," he said, "but I'll stake my wig there's fever here".

Robert Louis Stevenson, <u>Treasure Island</u>, (first published 1883)

Disease and Place

For centuries, cities were viewed as the natural sites of disease and corruption. High levels of mortality in the mushrooming metropoli of early modern and eighteenth-century Europe were expected, though deplored, as the result of too many people living in too small an area. As nineteenth-century American cities swelled with a steady stream of immigrants and the birth of industrialization, they also suffered from unsavory reputations and growing mortality rates.[1] Population density, combined with rudimentary or nonexistant methods of waste disposal, supported the prevailing theory that disease resulted from *miasmata* — a corruption of the air which produced a variety of illnesses.[2] This theory helped to explain the waves of epidemics which ravaged settled regions of the eastern United States, most catastrophic of which were the yellow fever outbreaks between 1793 and 1820, and the cholera epidemics which occurred between 1832 and 1866.[3] However, many non-epidemic ailments, such as rickets and tuberculosis, also throve in the increasingly crowded cities of the early nineteenth century.

People often left urban areas in search of health. Nineteenth-century tuberculosis sufferers took sea voyages or journeyed to mountains and deserts, seeking the pure air which they hoped would set them free from the disease.[4] Doctors prescribed vacations at the seaside for delicate middle class invalids. Rural and unsettled places were believed to offer the healthiest possible environment in which to live. The image of the sturdy pioneer partnered that of the purity of virgin wilderness.

11

Nonetheless, the romantic optimism of early western migrants was soon dashed. Upon leaving eastern settlements, travelers lost access to resources which supported urban sufferers and their families in times of ill-health. Medical practitioners, apothecary's shops, restful bedrooms and orderly domestic arrangements were left behind. Yet, diseases such as smallpox, malaria, tuberculosis, diphtheria, scarlet fever and typhoid followed the migrants west.[5]

In the nineteenth century, as in earlier periods, there was good reason to fear these ailments, because most people died of communicable diseases, rather than the chronic disorders more likely to kill their twentieth-century descendents.[6] And, although these ailments sometimes erupted in epidemics, European populations and their colonial relations had developed high levels of resistance to them, enabling many contagious diseases to become endemic. Thus, while Native American tribes invariably sustained devastating mortality after coming into contact with "European" diseases for the first time, pioneer carriers of these ailments suffered and sometimes died from them, but also established them in the areas they settled.[7]

Central Illinois had the reputation for being unusually unhealthy. Early nineteenth-century visitors remarked particularly on the fevers infesting the region. Although accurate diagnostic tests for the disease did not exist until the beginning of the twentieth century, most of the agues, chills, autumnal, bilious, remittent and intermittent fevers they reported were probably malaria. The disease was fostered by the environment, which was largely low, wet, and undrained, already inhabited by a large mosquito population which eagerly transported plasmodia from one human host to another. Settlers recognized an environmental cause for the fevers they experienced, but explained it in terms of the miasmas rising from newly broken virgin prairie soils or the amorphous dangers lurking in the night air. So common was intermittent fever that it was an expected part of life. Mrs. Tillson, recounting her experiences in Pike County in 1821, wrote, "An illness native in the prairie country was fever and ague. There was a burning fever following chills which left the patient so weak he could not work. It came with perfect regularity."[8] An early historian, Dr. E. Duis, indicates that McLean County residents also suffered:

> Great western waste of bottom land,
> Flat as a pancake, rich as grease;
> Where mosquitoes are as big as toads
> And toads are full as big as geese.

Beautiful prairie, rich with grass,
Where buffaloes and snakes prevail;
The first with dreadful looking face,
The last with dreadful sounding tail.

I'd rather live on a camel's rump
And be a Yankee Doodle beggar,
Than where they never see a stump
And shake to death with fever *ager*.[9]

Malaria, in addition to other fevers and fluxes, was popularly associated with "seasoning" — a phenomenon related to the process of adapting to new conditions, establishing a home and cultivating the soil. The settler's first season or two was often quite healthy, but once the land had been plowed, fever arrived. Dr. Duis also noted this phenomenon, writing

> The year 1831 was particularly celebrated for the fever and ague. A great deal of rich soil was turned over for the first time, and the vapors and exhalations made the climate unhealthy. . . . [Ague] was as much to be expected as harvest or the changes of the seasons.[10]

Dr. Daniel Drake of Cincinnati, who became the best informed expert of his day on the diseases of the midwest, had several correspondents in Illinois during the 1840s. One of them, Dr. John F. Henry, who lived in Bloomington between 1833 and 1843, was "convinced that an extensive plowing up of the soil of the prairies for the first time had been followed by fever."[11]

Other causes were also identified. Drake himself wrote:

> Its attacks are generally preceded by an exciting cause; such as irregularities in diet, or a debauch; above all, getting wet and cold, or sleeping exposed to the night air. A long ride through the dews of night or under the hot sun, of an early autumnal day, will alike excite it.[12]

Sufferers became depleted and depressed as the disease lingered. And, while the quinine they took for all fevers was actually effective in controlling the symptoms of malaria, the disease caused significant mortality in Illinois, which declined only with the draining and tiling of agricultural lands during the last half of the nineteenth century.

Malaria was particularly virulent during early years of settlement. As towns developed, other communicable diseases, including smallpox, typhoid, cholera, diphtheria, tuberculosis, diarrheal diseases and ailments now known to be caused by streptococci, including scarlet fever, erysipelas, and puerperal fever, increased in incidence.

Always endemic and sometimes epidemic in Europe and Africa, smallpox was an early import from the old to the new world. Although Jenner's vaccination technique was well known and accepted by the early years of the nineteenth century, many people remained unvaccinated. Thus, the new communities which developed in central Illinois displayed the familiar pattern of regular occasional incidence of the disease, interspersed at intervals with fierce and frightening epidemics. Their children, too, grew up with the threat contained in the traditional English dancing game:

> Ring a ring of roses
> A pocketful of posies;
> Ashes, ashes, we all fall down.

Smallpox was such a routine visitor to nineteenth-century Illinois that, apparently, in some areas unpocked faces were considered beautiful because they were so uncommon.[13] One of the few diseases generally assumed to be contagious, smallpox was feared out of all proportion to its danger. For example, in early Bloomington, Dr. Henry, mentioned above, took into his own home an eight-year-old girl and her mother who were suffering from smallpox to save them from being expelled from the settlement by the terrified residents.[14]

Even more feared than smallpox was Asiatic cholera, which first visited the United States in 1832. Although more devastating to eastern population centers, outbreaks also occurred in many parts of Illinois during that pandemic, returning at intervals until public health measures succeeded in fending off an epidemic in the 1890s.[15] Cholera struck and killed with lightning speed. Describing the 1849-52 outbreak in Henry County, one observer wrote, "Men would go to work in the morning in good health and be dead before sundown."[16] Thus, the disease terrified, even at a distance. Newspapers tracked its progress through neighboring areas. Communities cleaned their streets, banned the entrance of travelers from affected areas, and implemented a variety of public health measures in the hope of keeping it at bay.[17] Thus, even before identification of the means of transmission (1850s) or discovery of the cholera bacillus (1883), measures taken to prevent the disease worked — for the wrong reasons.

Not identified as a specific disease until 1829, typhoid was often confused with other fevers, including typhus (carried by lice), and malaria (sometimes called typho-malaria). Caused by water and milk supplies contaminated by human and animal wastes, typhoid was more common when people relied upon private wells and backyard privies than it became after installation of public sewage systems and water supplies. Because typhoid could be carried by a symptomless individual for years, it often appeared as an isolated incident, unrelated to specific local conditions or sources of contagion. In 1863, Dr. Harrison Noble reported to the State Medical Society, "Typhoid first came to McLean County in 1846 and 1847." In 1850, Bloomington's Dr. Roe wrote, "Typhoid fever is now first in importance. Perhaps not even cholera exceeds in the number of its victims this fell disease. It is almost as yesterday this disease made its first appearance among us."[18] Characterized by a rash, headache, abdominal pain, and bowel hemmorhages, typhoid inflicted on its victims a long-lasting fever, whose typical fluctuation from morning low to afternoon high gave it the name "snake fence".

More common and deadly than typhoid was diphtheria, often also reported as croup. A disease mainly afflicting children, it killed by obstructing the windpipe. Like smallpox, scarlet fever, measles, and whooping cough, diphtheria tended to be a constant presence, but flared up in devastating epidemics every few years. Although the diphtheria bacillus was identified in 1883, and antitoxin introduced in 1895, diphtheria continued to kill children in McLean County until the mid-twentieth century.

Tuberculosis was a leading killer in the United States for much of the nineteenth century, earning its popular soubriquet "the white plague". Until the tubercle bacillus was discovered by Koch in 1882, the disease was not generally regarded as contagious. Instead, many other causes were identified for what in its pulmonary form was usually called "consumption", including an inherited predisposition, too much brain work, licentious lifestyles, and unhealthy living conditions. Although it was generally believed that hard physical labor and fresh air were beneficial in the treatment of tuberculosis, involuntary outdoor therapy did not seem to prevent the disease among McLean County's early settlers: at least eight of the 78 deaths reported in 1850 were due to consumption, with the likelihood that five more attributed to ailments such as "inflamation of the lungs" and "lung disease" brought the real total to nearly 17 percent. Unlike many other communicable diseases which attacked and killed quickly, tuberculosis took a long time to consume its victims, stealing their energy and ability to function before taking their lives. It thrived in the crowded unsanitary living conditions of pioneer households, affecting the productivity of adult workers. It also complicated many pregnancies, thus inflating the number of postpartum deaths.[19] Although deaths from tuberculosis declined in Illinois communities toward the beginning of the twentieth century, the disease remained a significant killer until streptomycin was introduced in the late 1940s.

More dangerous than tuberculosis, typhoid or smallpox, but less feared, were the diseases characterized by diarrhea. Often associated with other ailments, such as malaria, typhoid, or cholera, "the flux" was not generally taken very seriously. However, diarrhea and dysentery were both common and deadly in early Illinois. Practitioners reported epidemics, which tended to occur in the late summer. Describing an outbreak of dysentery in LeRoy in 1860, a Dr. J.W. Coleman wrote "No class, age or sex were exempt. About one patient died out of each fifteen sick but five miles from LeRoy on the Bloomington road twenty cases developed of whom six died."[20]

Table 1

Death rates per 100,000 population from certain diseases in Illinois, 1860-1900[24]

	1860	1870	1880	1881	1882	1883	1884	1885	1890	1900
Malaria	66.9	35.5	36.1	23.8	11.3	11.3	10.8	11.2	19.1	10.3
Smallpox	0.4	6.7	1.4	54.6	81.8	3.1	.32	1.8	------	.51
Typhoid	65.7	70.3	53.6	66.0	44.1	31.9	31.5	39.9	44.4	39.3
Tuberculosis	113.7	145.6	150.9	111.7	73.8	98.5	102.5	111.9	148.9	140.7
Diphtheria	70.0	59.0	122.9	92.7	67.2	66.6	68.6	79.8	*93.0	42.8
Scarlet fever	98.7	85.1	44.4	27.1	21.2	31.7	24.6	23.2	11.5	13.3
Diarrheal diseases	128.8	188.3	148.0	181.5	107.7	109.7	110.0	106.5	------	----**
Pneumonia and Influenza	79.2	113.4	142.2	118.0	92.7	76.2	79.0	80.0	128.3	143.9

*This table does not include the year 1886, when the death rate from diphtheria reached 113.3.

**In 1902, the next year for which figures are available, the death rate from diarrheal diseases dropped to 79.5.

Diarrhea was particularly deadly among young children and, indeed, was a major cause of the high infant mortality rate which, in 1880 still hovered at approximately 200 per 1,000 births reported in Illinois.[21] Nearly half of all deaths reported in Bloomington in 1850 were among children under age five. Attributed to cholera infantum, cholera morbus, summer complaint, diarrhea, dysentery, or even teething, these deaths also tended to occur during the summer. Diarrhea and dysentery mystified the physicians of the time. Even Abraham Jacobi, founder of pediatrics as a medical specialty, believed that cholera infantum resulted from paralysis of the nervous system caused by heat. Many writers thought it was caused by malaria, and advocated using quinine to prevent its incidence.[22] Some advocated the use of emetics to prevent diarrhea.[23] However, only after popularization of the germ theory and associated changes in domestic hygiene in the early twentieth century did the number of deaths from diarrheal diseases decline.

Domestic Medicine

> Jack and Jill went up the hill to fetch a pail of water;
> Jack fell down, and broke his crown, and Jill came tumbling after.
> Then up Jack got and home did trot as fast as he was able.
> He went to bed and bound his head with vinegar and brown paper.
> *Traditional nursery rhyme*

What did McLean County residents do when they became ill? The answer to this question varies greatly depending on the time period, socio-economic class, and geographical location of the person concerned. Nonetheless, it is fair to say that for most people before about 1920, health care took place at home and was administered by women. Along with basic cooking, sewing and other housework, young girls traditionally learned how to prepare remedies and nurse the ailing. Older women became medical authorities within their families and communities, consulted for advice about health maintenance and disease prevention; infant and child care; pregnancy and birth; injury, illness and death.[25] Their knowledge was based on several traditions. Some health lore was semi-magical; some dependent upon a knowledge of herbs; some based purely on successful experience. All was taught within the family and nurtured by ongoing need.

Early McLean County residents had neither the same access to, nor the same expectations of medical practitioners which would develop among their descendents. They settled initially on farmsteads, isolated by distance, barriers to communication and the difficulty of travelling anywhere. There were no roads, no telephones. Even when doctors lived nearby, they were seldom conveniently available in an emergency. Furthermore, cash-poor farming families worried about the expense of paying a physician. Thus, people were forced by their living circumstances to depend upon family members and near neighbors when a health crisis arose. A dramatic example of self treatment appears in the reminiscence of John Berry Orendorff, born in 1827 in Blooming Grove:

> Major [Seth] Baker was a remarkable man. A true type of
> the early pioneers of Blooming Grove. He had a steady
> nerve with a wonderful will power, always ready and willing to face all obstacles. As proof of this . . . [I] will state
> one case — he had a very sore toe that was very painful to
> him. He couldn't get it to heal, so he decided the toe had to
> be cut off, but there was not a surgeon or surgeon's tools in
> McLean County. He asked several men to take a chisel and
> cut his toe off. They were all afraid to do it as he might
> bleed to death. He got his chisel, made a keen edge to it,
> placed his foot on a solid block of wood, then placed the
> edge of the chisel to the diseased toe, then one stroke with
> the mallet severed the toe from the foot. He dressed the
> wound and gave it close attention till it healed up, and that
> was sooner than anyone expected. I think that was the
> first surgical operation by white people at Blooming
> Grove.[26]

People making medical decisions and providing care relied primarily on a combination of expedience, personal experience, traditional lore, and reference to "the old-time family medicine book that along with the Bible used to be on the table of sitting rooms in many a home in the United States."[27]

In the mid-nineteenth century, McLean County families were able to choose from a wide variety of books providing medical instructions. Cookbooks routinely contained a few recipes for remedies. For example, *The Home Cook Book of Chicago* (1874), based on recipes provided by Illinois housewives, suggested the following treatments:

> FOR SORE THROAT. — Cut slices of salt pork or fat
> bacon; simmer a few moments in hot vinegar, and apply to
> throat as hot as possible. When this is taken off, as the
> throat is relieved, put around a bandage of soft flannel. A
> gargle of equal parts of borax and alum, dissolved in water,
> is also excellent to be used frequently.
> HEALING LOTION. — One ounce glycerine, one ounce
> rosewater, ten drops carbolic acid. This preparation prevents and cures chapping of the skin, and at the same time
> bleaches it. It is also excellent for sore lips and gums. . . .
> TO STOP BLEEDING. — A handful of flour bound on the
> cut. . . .
> TO RESTORE FROM STROKE OF LIGHTNING. —

Shower with cold water for two hours; if the patient does not show signs of life, put salt in the water, and continue to shower an hour longer.[28]

Many such works simply offered lists of both human and animal ailments, together with prescribed therapies. However, the expanding genre of books focused exclusively on home medical treatment tended to provide some information on anatomy and physiology, diagnostic methods, and therapeutic advice.[29]

Some of these works self consciously offered alternatives to the heroic medicine practised by many doctors, even attacking the profession for trying to mystify vulnerable lay people with complicated theories and long words. Others argued that physicians were largely unnecessary. Dr. Daniel H. Whitney, whose *The Family Physician and Guide to Health* was published in 1833, wrote:

> I have always been surprised to see people look with so much confidence to the physician, in cases of imminent danger, and place so much stress upon the necessity of his presence when all that he was doing or could do was to give an emetic, perhaps, or a dose of calomel. . . the practice of medicine is not of half the consequence that it is generally imagined to be.[30]

However, most works encouraged sufferers to consult doctors if possible, but to dose themselves, when professional help was unavailable, with the same violent purges, opiates, and metallic remedies which physicians generally prescribed. Thus, families kept a variety of conventional remedies on hand, usually including calomel, jalap, tartar emetic, ipecac, castor oil, laudanum, opium, and quinine. Adults (particularly women) developed a good working knowledge of what were thought to be appropriate doses of these powerful substances, and even as late as the 1920s were expected by physicians to mix their own compound prescriptions.[31]

Nonetheless, use of strong medicines sometimes had unintended consequences. According to an early settler, two Blooming Grove children, Omen and Catherine Olney, got "the itch" when very young. "Friends recommended Red Percipity. They used it, had to go out in the rain, got wet, both got deaf and Catherine lost her speech."[32] She lived into her late thirties, remaining a deaf-mute.

In addition to these medicines, which had to be supplied by

often distant pharmacies and paid for with scarce cash, McLean County residents made their own remedies. Many had learned the medicinal properties of a large variety of plants which were either cultivated for that purpose or grew wild in the fields and forests of the area. Like familiarity with pharmaceuticals, herb lore was shared by professional physicians and lay people. Thus, Dr. Silas Hubbard, who practiced in Hudson during the second half of the nineteenth century, paid local residents to gather the medicinal plants he used in his practice.[33]

People also made remedies from household ingredients. Every family had its favorite recipe for cough syrup. Goose grease and flannel cloth were applied to congested chests. Warm oil was poured into sore ears. Like Jack in the nursery rhyme, they plastered and comforted a bruise with vinegar and brown paper. Soap and sugar poultices were used to "draw" boils. Mustard plasters were used for pneumonia and other serious lung ailments. In the absence of bandaids and adhesive tape, people used fabric to bandage wounds. Obvious fractures were splinted; bleeding was stopped by a variety of mechanical and medicinal means.

Despite this arsenal of practical knowledge, little could be done to cure the army of diseases threatening early residents of McLean County. Nineteenth-century ailments, when they did not kill immediately, lasted a long time. Nursing was done at home, and it involved intense hands-on patient care. With no reliable weapon against fever, women spent long days and nights sponging and watching sufferers. Lacking the convenient pills and sweetened syrups of the modern pharmacopoeia, determined carers forced large quantities of foul-tasting medicinal draughts down unwilling throats. Without modern fabrics and washing machines, the struggle to keep patients clean was Herculean. Special meals demanded by custom and humoral tradition had to be prepared. In the small cabins first built by settlers, the ailing shared rooms and beds with the healthy. Often without recourse to a physician's presumed expertise, carers had to depend upon their own knowledge and skill, taking responsibility for all decisions and outcomes.

Despite their efforts, the outcome often was not good. Indeed, death was, in most cases, considered to be the "natural" consequence of many ailments and even certain times of life. Stillbirth and death in infancy or old age were so common that death certificates routinely recorded these conditions as the cause of death. Certain illnesses were regarded as incurable. Dr. William Matthews's *Treatise on Domestic Medicine*, published in Indianapolis in 1848, indicated that once consumption was "firmly fixed upon the lungs," the physician's main role was to ease the patient's death.[34] In early McLean County homes, the sick-bed often became the death-bed. The final service rendered by the mother, wife, servant or neighbor was often preparation of the victim's body for burial.

Calling the Doctor

When physicians were available and there were serious health problems, people called the doctor. They were, indeed, prepared to travel many miles under difficult conditions to obtain expert assistance. According to a late nineteenth-century local historian,

> In 1830 the doctors were not so numerous as at present. Young Esek [Greenman] remembers some horseback exercise when he rode to Pekin, a distance of thirty-three miles, wihout saddle or stirrups, for the doctor. On his return with the doctor he forded the Mackinaw on the upper side, so that, if swept from his horse by the current, the doctor could catch him.[35]

Because of their special skills and the hazards of pioneer life, surgeons were often in more demand than physicians. An early McLean County resident, John B. Orendorff, remembered a potentially disastrous childhood prank played by Simon Olney one Thanksgiving Day. Having been left alone with his younger siblings, Simon "decided to have some jolification":

> He got the powder flask and . . . commenced to sprinkle powder on coals that was scattered on the hearth and was having a gay time till he happened to extend his hand over the burning coals so the burning powder flashed in the flask. It went off and up through the ceiling with a crash and a report that was heard a long ways. It tore the thumb of his right hand so it was turned clear back on his wrist just like it had been cut with some sharp instrument. the thumb hung perfectly loose. They sent to Bloomington for Dr. Henry. He replaced the joint and sewed up the wound so it healed up in course of time, but his thumb was as stiff as a bone, couldn't bend it a particle.[36]

However, people also valued the services of physicians, whose effectiveness was often based upon long relationships with whole families. Orendorff remembered with fondness Dr. George Espy who began practice in Bloomington in the 1840s: [37]

Doctor Espy had a very extensive practice for a great many years, I think between 35 and 40 years. He was considered the leading doctor of Bloomington — was very successful in chills and fevers. . . . The night was never too dark or stormy for him to go, then he was very moderate in his charges. . . . He was our family doctor for a good many years. I remember well going after him one terrible stormy night for my mother that was suddenly taken ill with something like the bilious colic. All the home remedies were of no avail. Her suffering was terrible. We all felt very much alarmed about her — the nearest neighbor was a mile away. I was the oldest of the children, then 14 years of age. Father says to me, "Can you go after Doc Espy." I says yes. . . . In less than five minutes I was on my way. As I mounted my horse, Father says, "Berry, let your horse go, your Mother's life may probably be saved if you make good time."

In this case, the doctor was roused from his own sickbed and treated Mrs. Orendorff, who recovered.[38]

The same Dr. Espy was called to attend Mrs. Omen Olney, a "large muscular woman". . . who "weighed over two hundred pounds and was possessed of wonderful strength":

She had a hard spell of bilious fever for some time. She was not expected to live, but after lingering some four or six weeks between life and death, she took a turn to get well and gained very rapid so she was able to be about her household work again. But all of a sudden she became very weak and violently insane, and for six weeks she was a raving maniac. The doctor said the insanity was caused by her fever. They had to place a lock and chain to her ankle and with a staple fastened at the other end of the chain that was spiked to the floor. Also had her bedstead nailed to the floor. . . . One day while Dr. Espy was treating her at an unguarded moment, she gathered him and jammed him and his head under a forestick of a big burning fire into a red hot bed of coals and would have burnt him to death if some parties that was just coming in had not hastened to his relief and dragged him out of his perilous situation . . . . At the time she was insane we had no insane asylums to take the insane to. Don't think there was anything of the kind in the state at that time. After she became sane again, she then kept rational as long as she lived.[39]

Generally speaking, people did not expect doctors to cure them or their loved ones. However, they were consulted when all other means had been exhausted or when sudden illness appeared to be potentially fatal. Doctors were expected to have special knowledge of medical theories and therapies. They also were expected to assume some of the responsiblity for the patient, thus lightening the burden of relatives. To some extent, doctors were expected to look the part. They must radiate confidence; it helped if they were mature in years. Thus, young doctors began practice under a certain amount of suspicion. An account of the career of Dr. John M. Major, who practiced medicine in Bloomington between about 1849 and 1867 recalled:

> In January 1850, Dr. Parsons [Major's much older medical partner] was called to go twenty miles in the country, and, as he did not wish to face the intense cold, sent young Dr. Major. He gave the latter a letter of introduction to an old widow lady, whose children were very sick with pneumonia. Dr. Parsons had been the old lady's family physician, in whom she had great confidence, and she was much disappointed with the juvenile appearance of Dr. Major. ... But when this juvenile, adding a year or so to his age, told her he was twenty-five, she allowed him, with some misgivings, to prescribe for her children. He was successful in curing them, and she was quite as well satisfied as if the old doctor had been present, for she had thought it was age that made the doctor, and not the man.[40]

Then as now, demeanor and doctoring went hand in hand. The moral and emotional support nineteenth-century physicians gave patients and their families was, perhaps, both more important and more effective than the therapies they prescribed.

Pregnancy and Childbirth

Traditionally, pregnancy and birth were considered exclusively female matters — socially taboo, and outside the realm of the layman's knowledge or interest. Nineteenth-century culture forebade sex education of any kind. Modest women were expected to hide their naked bodies even from themselves. Thus, urban couples ("nice" girls, in particular) often went to their marriage beds completely ignorant about what was expected to take place, and equally often spent their adult lives without considering family planning a possible undertaking.[41] Pregnant women, whose participation in sexual activities was obvious, hid either their pregnancies or themselves from public view. Thus, both the weight of tradition and the force of contemporary mores made the birth chamber a female sphere. Traditionally , childbirth was managed by midwives, with the mother's female relatives and friends also in attendance.

However, by the nineteenth century, physicians had become increasingly interested in the practice of obstetrics for both professional and economic reasons. Unlike midwives, who used no instruments and few medicines, doctors had recourse to a variety of instruments, including forceps, and, by mid-century, anaesthetics. They were consulted by a growing number of women who hoped physicians could guarantee safer, speedier and less painful deliveries. The extent to which their hopes were justified is controversial among historians. Some historians argue that the growing tendancy for physicians to intervene in the birth process caused many postnatal problems among mothers, including tears, puerperal infection, and uterine prolapse. Others maintain that physicians became increasingly adept at repairing the damage done by botched deliveries, thus improving the quality of life for countless women.[42] Regardless, while midwives and nurses continued to manage births in McLean County throughout the nineteenth century, the physicians' sphere of influence grew, particularly in urban areas.

Nineteenth-century American women were often pregnant. Indeed, in 1800, white American women bore an average of more than seven live children, presumably undergoing several additional pregnancies ending in miscarriage or stillbirth. At the end of the century, this number had been reduced to an average of 3.56 babies; however, African-American women still bore an average of more than five children in 1900.[43] Thus, most women could expect to spend a significant portion of their adult lives either pregnant or recovering from childbirth. While many physicians regarded the "delicate condition" of nineteenth-century pregnancy as pathological, neither they nor midwives provided routine prenatal care. Pregnancy was guided by tradition and supported largely by female relatives and friends.

Before about 1920, like illness and death, virtually all births in McLean County took place at home. Indeed, until 1880, there were no hospitals in the county. Women sent for doctor, midwife, or nurse when labor approached, and gave birth in their own bedrooms, often with female friends or relatives also in attendance. There they stayed for the customary ten days or two weeks following delivery, since it was believed to be very dangerous for a woman to get up too soon. During this period, the housework and care of older children was done by female relations, friends, or hired nurses. Thus, regardless of who delivered the baby, the environment within which birth took place differed dramatically from that of the hospital deliveries which became customary during the next century. Home birth was governed by a combination of contemporary medical theory, tradition, and personal habits. Above all, it was controlled and managed by women and their families, rather than by professions and institutions.

Healing in McLean County: Doctors and Doctoring in the Nineteenth Century

The past is a foreign country. Despite universal human needs, past residents of the planet felt and acted differently from their descendants. Nonetheless, modern explorers of the past take with them many assumptions based upon their own experience and expectations, interpreting past experience according to current norms. This observation is especially significant regarding the history of professional medicine, because physicians have traditionally regarded themselves as direct heirs of past doctors, and medical historians have traditionally assumed the physicians' partisan and uncritical view of the historic doctor's role, motivation, status, and professional development. Thus, the tendency has been to chart the steady victory of the allopathic doctor-hero, who steadfastly fought a dual battle against disease and quacks, emerging triumphant in the twentieth century. While surviving evidence supports parts of this story, careful consideration also allows both a more ambivalent and a more interesting account of nineteenth-century doctors, doctoring, and the development of the medical profession.

Nineteenth-Century Healers and the Medical Scene

Unlike today's physicians, whose training, professional responsibilities, incomes and social status have become more or less standardized, nineteenth-century American doctors inhabited a broader spectrum of expertise, roles and rewards. They obtained their training in a variety of ways. The high-status physicians of eastern cities had degrees from the few universities offering medical programs, which were supplemented by training obtained in European universities, hospitals and laboratories. Indeed, many of these physicians were themselves Europeans — immigrants fleeing political unrest and seeking the opportunities offered by a young nation.

Elite physicians were the aristocrats of the profession, treating upper-class patients, commanding large fees, directing staffs of urban hospitals, teaching on university medical faculties, writing medical textbooks, and developing professional organizations. They agitated for higher standards in medical education, demanded legislation restricting practice to appropriately trained "regular" (allopathic) physicians, and attacked "irregulars" for charlatanism and endangering the bodies and purses of the gullible general public.

A more common preparation for medical practice was a combination of apprenticeship with a practicing physician, amplified by some classroom education in medical theory taken, more often than not, at a proprietary medical school (owned and operated by one or more physicians who taught all classes and pocketed all tuition payments). A usual career pattern was for a doctor to practice for several years between apprenticeship and academic training, sometimes interrupting classroom study to practice and earn before obtaining a medical degree.

In an age when most education was informal, there were no established standards for admission to the burgeoning number of medical schools. Toward the end of the century, most states began to require high school graduation as a prerequisite for entrance. However, there was little agreement about what constituted appropriate pre-medical education or, indeed, about the components of an appropriate medical school curriculum.

The quality of preparation provided by nineteenth-century medical schools thus varied enormously. A few offered a wide range of courses taught by experts in biological and physical sciences, attracting students who had no intention of becoming physicians, but who wanted to study science.[1] Others were less reputable, offering a small number of low quality courses and virtually selling diplomas. Medical schools provided few opportunities for clinical study, expecting students to obtain hands-on practical experience by assisting practicing doctors. So unreliable was the M.D. as an indicator of medical competence that in 1877 Illinois passed a law which empowered a board of medical examiners to deny doctors with diplomas from disreputable schools license to practice in the state.[2] Not until the early twentieth century would the Flexner Report stimulate reform and standardization of medical education based upon the Johns Hopkins model of laboratory-based academic course-work, taught by full-time faculty members and linked with a major university which conferred degrees.[3]

Rivaling allopathic medicine, which combined a new recognition of localism of disease in specific organs with traditional humoral therapeutic methods, a variety of medical sects propounding alternative theoretical and therapeutic approaches developed in nineteenth-century America.[4] Most influential was homeopathy, founded by the German Samuel Hahnemann, and embraced by some American physicians beginning in the 1820s. Based on the principal that "like cures like" (i.e., the idea of curing a disease with remedies which produced similar symptoms), and employing infinitesimal doses rather than the heroic draughts of the allopaths, homeopathy attracted both physicians and patients because it apparently did less harm than regular medicine. Homeopaths set up their own medical schools, dispensaries and pharmacies, by mid-century becoming significant rivals to regular physicians.[5]

Other early sects included Thomsonians, whose system of botanical medicine combined humoral theory with herbally induced therapeutic evacuation; hydropaths, who rejected professional medicine, substituting preventative measures which included intensive application of water internally and externally; and eclectics, who freely selected theories and therapies from other sects.[6] Later "irregulars" arriving on the medical scene in the 1890s were osteopaths and chiropractors, whose manipulative therapeutics were based on the premise that health and vigor depend upon correct alignment of the skeletal structure.[7] While osteopathy gradually incorporated many features of regular medicine, chiropractic remained unwilling to compromise its fundamental theoretical and therapeutic approaches.[8]

In addition to formal alternative practitioners, there were many unlearned healers offering their services to nineteenth-century Americans. Some of these were charlatans, selling sometimes dangerous remedies to members of a general public who were both gullible regarding the virtues of remedy and vendor, and skeptical concerning the superior abilities of physicians. This was the age of the medicine show, where patrons could be entertained and "cured" for the same small fee. Remedies were generally the vendor's own concoction, heavily alcohol-based, and promising to heal an improbable array of ills.[9] As demonstrated by Bloomington's own Dr. Cyrenius Wakefield, an ex-schoolteacher who became very successful in the patent medicine trade, regardless of training, virtually any man could call himself a doctor.[10]

However, not all unlearned practitioners were quacks. There were bonesetters, herbalists and barbers (who both pulled teeth and let blood), who developed a good deal of expertise and performed useful services. There were midwives, some well educated and formally trained, some depending entirely upon practical experience of attending many births. There were also many women who "developed considerable skill and perhaps science in the matter of treating the common ailments to which the flesh is heir." Such early Bloomington residents as Aunt Jane Hendrix, Aunt Ann Dawson and Mrs. Gardner Randolph used such therapies as "sweating and the use of native herbs" to treat their neighbors' ills.[11] According to one source:

> Mrs. Randolph . . . brought . . . an assortment of dried herbs, a bottle of Number Six — a villainous compound of pepper, camphor and other hot substances, administered in alcohol, and quite taking the skin off an ordinary throat, as I know to my sorrow — and the seeds of numerous other herbal remedies, such as thyme, madder, comfrey, elecampane, catnip, hoarhound and various other nauseous plants which spread over the neighborhood, and all of which she administered without stint or hesitation to such unfortunate victims as fell in her power. She was, besides, a notable midwife and rode on horseback for miles on the darkest nights to visit such families as needed her services.[12]

In addition to physicians, surgeons, quacks and unlearned healers, the nineteenth century witnessed the development of two medically related fields — dentistry and pharmacy. In traditional Europe, dentistry had been associated with barbering. Before the mid-nineteenth century, it had been taught exclusively by apprenticeship, and there was no regulation of the occupation. However, in the 1840s, its first professional school, the Baltimore College of Dental Surgery, was founded together with the American Society of Dental Surgeons.[13] Within a few years, American dentistry led the world, setting a standard for academic preparation and professional development unrivaled anywhere else.

Like dentistry, pharmacy was traditionally taught by practical rather than academic training. Due to the vogue for progressively more heroic treatment, which required larger quantities of drugs, the medicine trade became increasingly lucrative. With increasing possibilities in pharmacy based on developments in chemistry, the need for more sophisticated pharmaceutical training became apparent. The first American schools of pharmacy were founded in the 1820s.[14] However, during the nineteenth century, physicians and pharmacists remained competitors, since many doctors compounded and dispensed drugs, and many pharmacists provided diagnostic and therapeutic advice along with the remedies they sold.

In the early and mid-nineteenth century, the American people rejected as undemocratic attempts by physicians to regulate medical practice. Although local medical societies sprang up soon after settlement in most communities, and the American Medical

Association was founded in 1847 in order to raise the standards of medical practice and advocate the interests of allopathic physicians, early nineteenth-century attempts to obtain state licensing laws were stymied by egalitarianism, anti-monopolism, and suspicion of organized medicine. Rendered cynical by long exposure to heroic therapies and regular experience of death from virtually any cause, people rejected both the allopaths' claims to exclusive knowledge and their attacks on quacks, who turned out to be all non-allopathic practitioners. The public reserved the right freely to select healers and cures. Thus, the nineteenth century witnessed a free-for-all in America's medical marketplace.

There were lots of doctors to join in the fray. As proprietary medical schools became more numerous, making it easy for almost anyone to obtain a diploma, the number of M.D.s mushroomed. During the 1830s, allopathic medical schools graduated approximately 6,800 physicians, the number of graduates rising to nearly 18,000 in the 1850s.[15] Eastern markets were saturated. Medical graduates were encouraged to go west. An 1854 contributor to the *Boston Medical and Surgical Journal* wrote:

> Why not strike manfully into the virgin regions of the West, and grow up with society [there], into wealth, usefulness and distinction? . . . Wherever there are human beings, there the advice of the physician is required; and as population increases, so does the odor of his good name. In short, prosperity and usefulness will in most cases be the reward of those who leave the old hive, to act their parts and gather and get gain in the unoccupied localities of Oregon, Nebraska, and Kansas.[16]

Doctors and Doctoring in Early McLean County

West they came, some of them settling in McLean County. The 1850 Census lists sixteen men identifying themselves as doctors. While some of these may not have been active practitioners, and others not formally qualified M.D.s, by modern standards, this was a very large number for a community totaling only 1,594.[17]

What were the lives of these early physicians like? Doctors Henry and Conkling provide examples of typical nineteenth-century medical biographies, including the combination of apprenticeship, practice before achievement of the M.D., and experience of a variety of careers in addition to medicine. Dr. Thomas Rogers' day books offer a glimpse of the typical day-to-day working life of a mid-nineteenth-century physician.

Dr. J.F. Henry

Dr. John Flournoy Henry was born to a well-to-do Kentucky family reputed to be of Huguenot ancestry. Born in Henry's Mills, Scott County, Kentucky in 1793, he began the study of medicine as a teenager and served as surgeon's mate during the War of 1812. He undertook an academic course at the College of Physicians and Surgeons in New York City, receiving his diploma in 1818. Serving briefly as a Congressman in 1826, where he filled a vacancy created by his brother's death, he also practiced medicine in Kentucky and worked as a professor at the Ohio Medical College in Cincinnati. In 1833, Dr. Henry settled in Bloomington, where he practiced medicine for twelve years and became a regular correspondent of Dr. Daniel Drake, informing him about local health conditions.[18] In 1845, he moved to Burlington, Iowa, shortly thereafter retiring from practice, having "secured a competency" (i.e., become sufficiently wealthy to stop working). Dr. Henry died in Burlington in 1873. He was described by a contemporary as:

> one of nature's noblemen. Tall and straight as an arrow, with a splendid presence and a physical vigor, which is rare in these latter days of fast habits and rapid living; he enjoyed a robust health . . . . He was a fine specimen of the Kentucky gentleman of the old school, of elegant and dignified manners, kindly sentiments and genial disposition.[19]

Dr. Henry Conkling

Dr. Henry Conkling was born in Morristown, New Jersey, in 1814. Receiving his basic education at the Morristown Academy, he emigrated to Mt. Vernon, Ohio, in 1832. He married there at age 23, then decided to move further west, traveling on horseback the distance to Leroy, in McLean County, in 18 days. Having settled there, he taught school and studied medicine with Dr. David Edwards, an established practitioner. In 1843, he began to practice independently, offering his services first in Mount Hope, then in Washington. In 1845, he returned to Ohio where he practiced while studying at the Starling Medical College of

Columbus. Returning to McLean County in 1850, he practiced first in Hudson, then in Bloomington, before serving as a surgeon in the Union army. Beginning in 1866, he became involved in plans to construct a railroad line from Danville through Bloomington to the Illinois River. Until 1870, this project was his primary activity. Thereafter, he became proprietor of the Turkish and Electro-Thermal Institute in Bloomington, which offered hydrotherapy both to invalids and those who took the baths as a luxury.[20]

Dr. Thomas Pierce Rogers

What were the working lives of early McLean County physicians like? The day books kept by Dr. Thomas P. Rogers between 1839 and 1854 offer a window through which to observe their daily activities.[21] Rogers was born in 1812 in Ohio. His medical training came via practical study with a doctor in Tuscarawas County, Ohio, completed by an academic course in Philadelphia.[22] He began practice in Decatur in 1838, moving to Bloomington in 1849 because he learned that the Illinois Central Railroad was likely to run through the town. Although medical fees in his day were not large, Dr. Rogers attracted a large and loyal clientele. He became prosperous, retiring in 1867 at the age of 55 to "engage in agricultural pursuits."[23] He also became active in politics, serving in the state legislature in the 1870s.

With the exception of the last five years, Rogers' day books were written when he was practicing in Decatur. Thus, strictly speaking, they mainly document the treatment of Macon County residents. However, the doctor's therapeutic approach, routines and charges were the same after his move to Bloomington as they had been in Decatur. Thus, they provide a useful early source of information about these matters.

Although Dr. Rogers had a series of professional partners (who presumably offered cover during high volume periods or absences) and kept an office, he spent much of his time making house calls. His pattern was to visit patients at least once a day during the course of their illnesses. Dr. Rogers dispensed, and probably mixed, the remedies he prescribed. Most of the clients who visited his office apparently came to purchase medicines.

Rogers' day books do not provide information about symptoms or diagnoses. Rather, they record the names, genders and, sometimes, ages of patients; remedies and services provided; and fees charged. Most of Rogers' business was what would now be called internal medicine. Prescriptions indicate that he treated many fevers, chest infections and gastrointestinal upsets. His approach was typical of allopaths of his day, depending upon evacuation in the form of laxatives, emetics and blood-letting to restore his patients' humoral balance. Frequently repeated medical ingredients include senna, castor oil, antimony, cream of tartar, camphor and calomel, in addition to unspecified tonics, bitters, cathartics and pills. Rogers sold patent remedies, including Doverspowder and Rockwell salts. He also prescribed opiates under a variety of circumstances and a great deal of quinine for fever. He let blood, sometimes as part of a treatment regimen, sometimes prophylactically. In addition to practicing internal medicine, Rogers treated skin diseases, pulled teeth and delivered babies.

Although the doctor became a wealthy man, his charges for individual services were modest. House calls in town cost $1.00; rural and night visits added to the fee. For instance, for a night journey of nine miles in January, 1840, he charged the patient's husband $7.00, which included medications (an emetic and "oil"). Canny clients often asked him to treat more than one patient in the household during a single visit, thus incurring only a single charge for the call. Rogers charged fifty cents for simple tooth extractions and $5.00 to deliver babies.

Despite his very moderate fee scale, Rogers' patients spent a good deal of money for medical care because of its labor-intensive nature. Nineteenth-century disorders tended to linger; Rogers made frequent visits to his patients during the course of their illnesses. Thus, patients tended to run up substantial tabs, which Rogers charged monthly. Mr. Charles Baker incurred charges of $22.50 for nearly daily attendance during September of 1851 — a sum which seems ludicrously small today, but which was considerable by the standards of the time.

Thomas Rogers' financial and professional success owed more to his political and business talents than to the economic potential of nineteenth-century medical practice. In cost-benefit terms, doctoring in the period was an inefficient and uncomfortable route to prosperity. Physicians worked very long hours and faced daunting environmental hazards, including exposure to the gamut of nasty communicable diseases and to the difficulties of rural travel. Without surprise, one local historian remarks of two of McLean County's early medical settlers, "Dr. Haines died in 1838 and Dr. Anderson in 1842, both believed to have succumbed to overwork in the hard conditions and much sickness of the time."[24] Dr. Parke (1823-1908), a Bloomington physician, remembered of his early years of practice:

> One great difficulty the pioneer doctor had to contend with in traveling over the prairie was the absence of land marks — so much sameness. Then, again, at certain times great districts in the neighborhood of sloughs were enshrouded in dense fog, making it impossible to locate one's self, especially at night. Every pioneer medical man had more or less of this experience. During a practice of fifty years in McLean County I was lost three different times and wandered around until day-light, frequently was obliged to alight and feel for the roads, especially when riding a livery horse — they will invariably take to the grass when given the reins. The doctor's usual mode of travel in those days was on horseback with saddle-bags strapped on behind the saddle.[25]

Notwithstanding the challenges of professional life, physicians were respected members of nineteenth-century communities, remarkable for their comparatively advanced educations and their willingness to take on civic and business responsibilities. Thus, it is not surprising that doctors such as Rogers, Henry and Conkling left medical practice to become involved in railway projects, farming and politics. After the rigors of doctoring, these alternatives must have appeared safer, easier and far more lucrative.

Professional Life: the McLean County Medical Society

Incorporated in1843, between 1850 and 1870 Bloomington's population increased from 1,594 to 14,590. These were boom years, during which the Chicago and Alton Railroad works (established in 1853) became the area's primary employer[26,] Illinois Wesleyan University (founded in 1850) and Illinois State University (founded in 1857) became major educators in the state; and the Western Union Telegraph Company linked McLean County with the rest of the world (*circa* 1853). As the county became urbanized, medical practitioners followed the national trend by establishing the McLean County Medical Society in 1854.[27]

Only rudimentary records survive of the Society's first 37 years in existence.[28] However, records kept by the Society for the years between 1891 and 1910 provide a detailed account of its activities during that period. It is apparent that its members cultivated links with other county medical organizations and with the Illinois State Medical Society (founded in 1850). Although the McLean County Medical Society's constitution contains no mission statement, it is apparent from other sources that its primary purposes were to:

•regulate the local practice of medicine by excluding from its ranks irregular practitioners and "quacks";

•facilitate communication among local allopaths regarding scientific innovations, therapeutic controversies and local cases of interest;

•support progressive sanitary measures in the county (as long as these were controlled by physicians);

•and create a congenial forum for professional consultations, social activities and support of members and their families in times of hardship.[29]

From the beginning, the Society was open to allopaths conforming to a rarely articulated, but well understood code of professional behavior and ethics. They were not to advertise their services, either in newspapers or by other means. They must not prescribe or consult with practitioners offering cures associated with irregular practice. They must not sell or publically endorse patent or proprietary medicines. They must not poach each other's patients. The Society established a standard list of fees for the services most commonly offered, which individual practitioners ignored at their peril. Violations of these rules resulted in exclusion.

How did a medical practitioner become a member of the McLean County Medical Society? It apparently went without saying that applicants with degrees from reputable medical schools would be admitted once their credentials had been checked. However, the Society's constitution provided for the annual election of three Censors whose duty it was "to examine such applicants for membership as are not graduates in medicine and report to the society upon their qualifications for membership." Such a person was required to satisfy "the Censors that he has faithfully persevered in the study of medicine at least three years, and that he intends honestly and honorably to pursue the calling of his profession."[30]

Because members were determined to close ranks against alternative practitioners and quacks, discussion of whether or not to admit an applicant sometimes became heated and acrimonious. For instance, in September 1891, Dr. Homer Wakefield was proposed for membership. His mentor was Dr. James Branch Taylor, an early local specialist in eye, ear, nose and throat whose very respectable qualifications included graduation from the College of Physicians and Surgeons in New York City and attendance at medical lectures in Leipzig, Germany. Wakefield had made the mistake of advertising his services in the local newspaper. He also almost certainly suffered from the fact that his father, "Doctor" Cyrenius Wakefield, had established a very profitable patent medicine factory in Bloomington, likely earning both the envy and the contempt of the official medical establishment. The Society's Censors made a thorough check of Homer Wakefield's credentials, which resulted in the following drastic action:

> [At the November meeting], Dr. Little read a letter from Dr. Austin Flint, secretary of Bellevue Hospital Medical College of which school H. Wakefield is a graduate. He stated that Dr. Wakefield's name would be dropped from the Alumni Catalogue and that he had no suspicion Dr. Wakefield would become a quack.[31]

Dr. Taylor was enraged. In May of 1892, he refused to serve on the Society's banquet committee with Dr. Anderson, who had blocked Wakefield's admission, stating that "Dr. Wakefield, a student of his, was refused admittance into this the McLean County Medical Society on account of his newspaper advertisement and claiming that Dr. Anderson was equally as guilty in advertising his Keely Cure for drunkenness." At this point, Dr Hill accused Dr. Taylor, both of advertising and of consulting with a homeopath. Apparently, the matter was amicably resolved, since Dr. Taylor remained a member of the Society. However, it is unclear whether Homer Wakefield was ever admitted to membership, since his name does not appear among regular members in the organization's *Biographical History*, where it is only noted that in 1934 he was living in New York.[32]

In addition to its concern about the threat posed by local charlatans, the Society was also active in state-wide efforts of allopaths to block regulation of the practice of osteopathy. According to a Springfield newspaper quoted at a meeting in June 1897, the Governor had vetoed a recent bill on the grounds that it would open the door in Illinois "to incompetent, dishonest and unscrupulous adventurers calling themselves practitioners of osteopathy and there would be no remedy." The Society was still opposing passage of a similar bill in 1909.

Although the Society reserved membership exclusively for allopaths, it was apparently open-minded about gender and race, admitting appropriately qualified women and African Americans.

Doctors Rhoda Galloway Yolton and Eliza Hyndman were active members, Dr. Yolton serving as both secretary and president of the organization, while Dr. Hyndman served as its secretary. Dr. E.G. Covington, an African American, was admitted to the Society in 1901 without any mention of his race. Nonetheless, it is obvious that he mainly treated black patients. For example, in February 1908, he complained to the Society that some white physicians were charging "colored families who are able to pay the regulation fee of $2 per call . . . but $1.50 per visit. This, he says, works a hardship on him, as he is dependent mainly on the colored people for his living." The Society found in Dr. Covington's favor, condemning the lower charge. Nonetheless, Dr. Covington apparently became disaffected from the organization, being suspended from membership in 1910 when he had failed to pay his dues for two years.

Participation in the Society was extremely useful to members. They had access to ongoing professional development in the form of lectures given at monthly meetings by fellow members and guests. They developed invaluable relationships supporting consultations and referrals. As hospitals were built beginning in the 1880s, membership opened the door to hospital privileges. For newcomers to the county, membership validated qualifications and facilitated development of a clientele. Finally, the Society performed for doctors many of the functions labor unions offered to manual workers, protecting members in malpractice suits, protecting their incomes, discouraging competition from outsiders, including families in social activities and offering professional and financial assistance in times of illness and death.

Lectures delivered at monthly meetings served several purposes, allowing new members to demonstrate their abilities, giving established members a forum for their ideas and offering the membership as a whole the opportunity to keep abreast of changes in medical science and public health. These lectures exposed local practitioners to medical developments in other parts of the world. For instance, on May 6, 1897, Dr. John L. White "gave a very interesting talk on sanitary conditions in California cities Oakland and Alameda." In February 1899, Dr. T.W. Bath, Acting Assistant Surgeon with the U.S. army, gave a talk entitled "Some Observations on the Medical Conditions of Camp Life" in Cuba. In May, 1907, Dr. R.A. Noble discussed the question, "Is a Trip to Europe Worth its Cost to A Medical Man," reaching an affirmative conclusion and speaking favorably of the thoroughness and importance given in Germany to research work.

Lectures also encouraged members to talk about medical and surgical controversies of the day. In July 1897, after a paper given on "Conservatism in Surgery," there was heated discussion of appendectomy — a procedure introduced in the 1880s.[33] The speaker, Dr. White, contended that appendicitis was the fashionable disease of the day, and that many needless operations were performed. Dr. Rhoda Galloway Yolton then read a paper urging conservatism in the treatment of fibroid uterine tumors, broadening the discussion. Dr. Lee Smith "facetiously remarked that it was rather an unusual thing that two surgeons should at one time get together to give surgery a general scouring." Dr. Mammen contended that conservatism was sometimes fatal to the patient, and that the surgeon's duty was "to properly educate the public when surgery was necessary." Dr. Taylor argued that the trend of the future was for higher quality of work, while Dr. Little said that "too much eagerness to operate brings odium on the profession."

Lectures were used to introduce scientific and technological innovations in medicine. For instance, in January 1898, Dr. Eliza Hyndman gave a paper entitled "Some Aids in Diagnosis," which advocated a closer union of laboratory and clinical methods in diagnosis. On similar lines, in February of 1907, Dr. Ezra R. Larned of the Experimental Department of Parke, Davis & Company offered a lecture, illustrated with stereopticon slides, on the "Practical Application of Bacteriology to the Cure of Disease." In June 1903, a presentation on the "Use of the X-Ray for Diagnostic Purposes" was given. While decrying the apparently widespread and inappropriate use of x-rays by quacks, the speaker concluded that, "This form of electricity . . . is of inestimable use in diagnosing fractures, dislocations and in locating foreign bodies." X-Rays were also deemed to be useful in treating malignant disease, although this form of treatment should not be substituted for surgery in operable cases.

Medical Society records indicate the extent to which physicians took a leadership role in public health matters. For example, in 1897, there was great concern about the sanitary condition of Bloomington. The Society resolved "that all garbage, offal and rubbish should be taken beyond the city limits and burned." It advised the city government that "a garbage and offal crematory should be purchased and put in operation as soon as possible." Since the Society was still campaigning for the crematory in April of 1906, it is apparent that the city was not enthusiastic about this project.

Along the same lines, in May 1908, the Society called attention to the role of the common house fly in spreading disease. Dr. Vandervort stated:

> The season of the fly is approaching. Two things are necessary for the propagation and sustenance of the fly, . . . hot weather and filth. The first we cannot prevent and the latter we should fight against with all our might. As much garbage as possible should be burned by the housekeepers. Then the refuse should be carted away as soon as possible. The chief weapon that suggests itself against the fly evil is absolute cleanliness in the streets and houses and wherever there can be breeding places for the fly and the general use of screens. A careful houswife will never let a fly remain in the house. The experiences with typhoid fever in the camps of our soldiers during the Spanish American War demonstrated in a most forcible manner that the fly must be taken into consideration in fighting typhoid fever.

Physicians were active in campaigns for pure public water supplies, particularly when water-bourne diseases threatened. In January 1903, the Society reported on the incidence of typhoid fever in Bloomington during the past year. They contended that half of the 130 cases could be traced to the use of well water and that, although 18 patients used city (public) water, infection was almost certainly due to other sources. Thus, they advocated the use of city rather than private water supplies.

Physicians also were asked to offer advice about methods of dealing with infectious diseases. For example, in early 1907, the Medical Society formed a committee to confer with the school board regarding the length of time a child who had suffered an infectious disease should be kept at home. "It was the opinion of the committee that two weeks should be the minimum length of time at which the patient or other members of the family should be allowed to return to school after the discharge of said patient by his physician." The Society also became actively involved in the campaign to control tuberculosis, advocating the construction of sanitoria which could both offer treatment to sufferers and protect the healthy from infection.[34]

Society members were pleased to be consulted about civic policies regarding disease control, but were adamantly opposed to non-physicians having a role in public health measures involving direct contact with patients. Authority in medical matters and personal relationships with patients comprised the basis of their professional status and incomes. Anything infringing on that authority and relationship threatened their position. Thus, in May of 1891, Dr. Hill read the following resolutions at the monthly meeting:

> Whereas: The City Council of Bloomington making it obligatory for practicing physicians to report all cases of diphtheria to the health officer, therefore be it resolved that this society deprecates the practice of this City in sending its emissaries to the sick chamber to examine the case and decide as to its nature, prescribe and proscribe as suits him best in the absence of the attending physician. Also resolved that while we are willing to aid in all proper means to prevent the spread of contagious diseases, we as practicing physicians of this city and county protest against such undue interference with our private patients and practice.

It is not surprising that in April of 1897 the Society appointed a committee to advocate the appointment of a physician for Chief of the Bloomington Health Department.

Then as now, an important role the Society undertook was to support physicians in malpractice cases. The State Medical Society established a fund to help members pay legal fees, and the McLean County Medical Society discussed this fund and malpractice accusations in general at a meeting in October, 1907. According to the speaker, suits could be divided as follows: "50 percent are pure blackmail; 25 percent sue for malpractice to beat a just bill; 15 percent believe they have been aggrieved or injured; 10 percent are very close to malpractice. Blackmailers are generally charity patients." The speaker said that physicians "are loose in their methods of keeping books, frequently omitting dates and failing to make charges or record in their books of work done." He advised members to "keep a record of all cases." While no local malpractice cases are recorded, and malpractice insurance was a twentieth-century development, nineteenth-century Society members feared accusation and discussed ways of protecting themselves.

The Society was also active in regulating medical finances. While according to one presidential address in May, 1903, the Society's standard fee bill was not to be considered in the same light as an official wage scale, but merely as a guide for medical charges; nonetheless, this bill was obviously accepted as the basis for routine charges. It was renegotiated several times between 1891 and 1910, and doctors complained to the Society if their colleagues undercharged.[35]

In addition, the Society consistently opposed its members accepting the paid position of physician to any organization or agreeing "to do any medical or surgical work for any club, society or organization at a less rate than the regular customary charges for like services rendered by other physicians for patients not members of such a club, society or organization."[36] In October 1907, Dr. F. H. Godfrey in his presidential address discussed "the degrading effect of contract practice, citing . . . certain fraternal societies in which whole families receive medical treatment for 12 cents per week." In light of the contemporary international movement, best exemplified in Germany and Britain, favoring national insurance, the McLean County Medical Society provides an interesting example of the dominant opinion in American health care supporting private fee for service provision.

Alternative Practice

The records of the McLean County Medical Society provide a good deal of information about allopathic "regular" physicians. They also offer details about the Society's policies of excluding "irregular" practitioners; opposing state efforts to regulate alternative practices (notably osteopathy); and attempting to keep charlatans from working in McLean County. In 1898, for example, the Society met with Dr. Fox, a representative of the State Board of Health, who solicited its members' cooperation "concerning the intended prosecution of irregular practicing doctors in the City." In 1902, the Society formed a committee on Law to consider "the matter of flagrant abuses of their privileges among itinerant and irresponsible practitioners" considered to be "violators of law and decency."

In some cases, such actions were directed against the misinformation and harm which might be inflicted by irregulars on members of the unwary public. Thus, in 1908 the society called a special meeting "to take some action concerning certain erroneous remarks which have been made by one Flynn and his associate, Miss McIntire, who have been holding meetings in the churches of the city." Flynn was apparently billed as a lecturer on hygiene and a teacher of gymnastics. The Society decided to "draw up resolutions denouncing Flynn and present same to the Ministerial Association." In other instances, however, the Society appears to having been protecting its professional and financial interests. For example, in April of 1898, the Society:

Resolved that it is the sense of the members of the McLean County Medical Society in annual meeting assembled that it is clearly a violation of the code of Medical Ethics of the American Medical Association by which we profess to be guided and governed for any member of this Society to associate himself with an irregular advertising quack doctor for the purpose of carrying on and managing a Free Clinic such as the one which is located at no. 106 W. Monroe Street this City.

Regardless of the Society's power over medical practice in the area, however, a number of alternative practitioners established themselves in McLean County. Homeopaths began arriving in the 1850s. According to one source, there were nine homeopathic physicians practicing in Bloomington in 1908.[37] Two of these, Doctors George and Annie Kelso, opened their own hospital, the Kelso Sanitarium, in 1894. Specializing in surgery, diseases of women, chronic and nervous diseases and obstetrical cases, the hospital grew to include 60 beds and remained open until it was sold to the Mennonite Sanitarium Association in 1920.[38]

In addition to the homeopaths, an osteopathic physician, Dr. Boyle, began practicing in Bloomington in 1898, where he was joined by a number of colleagues in the early twentieth century. Chiropractors also appeared in the County soon after the establishment of their craft at the turn of the century. A Christian Science practitioner, Mrs. Della Rigby, arrived in Bloomington in about 1887 and, by 1908, had been joined by six more full-time practitioners and perhaps twelve who practiced part-time . In addition, "The city has also had its proportion of eclectic physicians. It has been a favorite resort for visiting specialists, and if McLean County has not been healthy, it has not been from lack in the multitude of its medical counselors."[39] Thus, although the County was dominated by allopathic physicians, who have also left the best records about their experience, it was also typical in supporting a multitude of alternative practitioners.

Conclusions

In the course of the nineteenth century, McLean County was transformed from a pioneer settlement on the fringe of American territory and society to an important social and commercial city in a major state. Provision of health care changed along with the population it served. Medical Society records illustrate the professionalization of allopathic physicians in the county. Urbanization brought the establishment of many dentists, pharmacists and trained midwives in the area. While most illnesses continued to be suffered and treated at home, the end of the century witnessed the establishment of hospital care.

By the end of the nineteenth century, popular expectations of official medicine were changing. While Pasteur and Lister had begun laboratory and empirical studies establishing the germ theory during the middle of the century, popularization of that theory really began in the 1880s and 1890s. Identification of specific microorganisms causing specific diseases, together with development of antitoxins which could cure or prevent some of those diseases, inaugurated an unparalleled sense of hope and power. For the first time, people began to believe they could defeat humanity's oldest enemy — death. Physicians, as the front-line representatives of scientific progress, were given credit for this progress. They began to accrue a cultural authority they had never had before. By 1906, the McLean County Medical Society was so secure in its position that it met amicably with local homeopaths and dentists. Doctors had gained what they had sought for at least 400 years — a virtual monopoly over the provision of medical care.

Despite advances in biomedical science and surgery, however, physicians and sufferers alike remained helpless in the face of major killers including most communicable diseases, cardiovascular illness and cancers. More significant than medical progress in the fight against disease were sanitation, drainage and general improvements in diet and housing.

Cleanliness is Next To Godliness: Public Health and Personal Hygiene

An Ounce of Prevention

In McLean County, as in other parts of the United States, mortality rates from most causes declined and life expectancy increased dramatically between 1830 and the present, with those changes escalating in the twentieth century. Although exact figures are not available, according to one source, "In the pioneer days in Illinois, few men were over 40 years of age. Men 50 years of age were regarded as old."[1] Another indicates that, "In 1900, life expectancy at birth was about 47 years. The life expectancy at birth in 1989 was 75 years of age."[2] Why did these changes occur? Although medical practitioners, particularly in the twentieth century, have developed ways of prolonging life which have made significant contributions, the greatest debt is owed to prevention activities, both personal and collective. Like medical therapies, these activities became much more effective after the popularization of the germ theory around the turn of the century. However, even before that time, personal hygiene and public health measures helped to save lives.

Private and public efforts to maintain health and prevent disease were not new in nineteenth-century America. Indeed, prevention was traditionally viewed as the best way of dealing with the threat of illness. Published works on the rules for maintaining good health are as old as the printing press.[3] Early diaries record the personal "regimens" followed by people who had experienced illness and wished to retain or regain their health.[4] Generally understood rules for healthy living supply the basis for personal and household management in any age.

They also underlie collective responses to epidemics. Although the means of transmission of diseases such as smallpox, plague and yellow fever were differently understood in traditional Europe and early America than they are today, it was obvious that these ailments were spread from one person to another. Thus, towns and cities strove to isolate sufferers in their own homes, in "pesthouses" or, in the case of travelers, outside of communities. Quarantines were enforced, either officially or informally, by residents terrified of becoming ill themselves.

In addition, cities threatened by epidemics initiated clean-

45

up campaigns to get rid of the garbage and human and animal waste from which dangerous *miasmata* were thought to emanate. For example, after 1832 repeated threats of cholera epidemics spurred the development of public health policies and structures in many American cities.[5] Such measures helped to make cities healthier places to live, regardless of whether the theories they were based on were "correct".

Technology has had an enormous impact upon health. Innovations such as field drainage tiles, the flush toilet, water purification, and pasteurization have undoubtedly saved more lives than antibiotics. Automobiles, while creating a variety of new dangers, have certainly reduced the hazard of widespread animal waste in the streets. Increasingly effective means of sterilizing baby bottles have decreased infant mortality from diarrheal diseases. Invention of disposable sanitary napkins and tampons have freed modern women from centuries of isolation, shame and inconvenience during menstruation. Today's mass-produced washable textiles, automatic washing machines, and indoor plumbing allow people to expect and take for granted a standard of personal cleanliness which would have been impossible for their nineteenth-century forebears. Thus, twentieth-century expectations of duration and quality of life owe a great deal to developments far removed from biomedicine.

Personal Hygiene

All deliberate efforts to maintain health and prevent illness are based upon the dominant medical theories of an era. Like the therapies of the period, nineteenth-century personal hygiene depended upon a combination of popular customs, humoral theory and newer organ-centered ideas about human physiology. Thus, while the conventional advice regarding moderation in diet sounds quite "modern", it actually was related to humoral injunctions against surfeit (which imbalanced the body's humors) and the notion that improper eating habits clogged the digestive passages, impeding efficient gastrointestinal functions. According to Catharine Beecher's *Letters to the People on Health and Happiness*, published in 1855:

> There is no way in which children have their stomachs weakened so frequently as by irregular and frequent eating. None of the muscles of the body are taxed so severely as those of the stomach, and they need periods of rest. If,

therefore, there is a constant entrance of food into the stomach, there is no time for rest, while there is a constant mixture of partly-digested and newly-arrived food that interrupts the natural process of digestion. From two to three hours pass before the stomach ceases its muscular action, and then it needs two or three hours to rest. The meals, therefore, should be five or six hours apart for grown persons.[6]

Beecher believed that adults of her time ate far too much and wrong-headedly devoured the most unhealthful foods available. She also argued against contemporary women's fashions which constricted the rib cage and abdomen, claiming that tight lacing impeded digestion, undermined the skeleton and threatened successful reproduction.

Nineteenth-century experts agreed that good health depended upon good diet, then, as now variously defined.[7] It also resulted from physical exercise in the open air. Thus, educators increasingly viewed a combination of mental and physical exercise as desirable for both boys and girls.

Fresh air itself was regarded as necessary for health. Houses were designed to promote good ventilation and keep bad air (i.e., sewer gas) below ground floor or street level. In addition, in an era before central heating, some forms of heating were regarded as healthier than others. Beecher argued that:

Open fire-places, that make a constant draught of the air of a room upward and outward, insure a constant supply of fresh air from the doors and windows. But close stoves, with tight doors and windows, make it almost certain that the inmates of a room will constantly breathe impure air, which will act as a slow poison in undermining the constitution. . . . And the richer our people grow the tighter they make their doors and windows, and the more they multiply stoves in sitting and sleeping rooms, and the less they exercise in pure air. While in some wretched country hovel the poor drink abundantly the life-inspiring and pure breath of heaven every hour of the day and night, the children of wealth sip it only for an hour or two, as they ride abroad in their luxurious equipages for "exercise and air."[8]

Experts of the time disagreed about the value and effects of bathing. Since, for most people, indoor plumbing was a late nineteenth- or early twentieth-century innovation, total immersion of the body was extremely inconvenient. Tub bathing involved transporting and heating large quantities of water, which must then be carried and disposed of once the bath was over. Since houses lacked bathrooms, in an excessively modest age privacy was also an issue. Thus, many families, if they bathed at all, made the effort only once a week or even less frequently.

Inconvenience notwithstanding, health issues associated with bathing were a matter of debate. For certain categories of people, including menstruating women and the physically weak, bathing was thought to be dangerously debilitating. Warm water, in particular, was frowned upon, while progressive thinkers favored cold. Catharine Beecher argued that, "A person in good health may take a cold bath every day, and gain vigor. But if he should take a hot bath as often and as long, it would debilitate. . . . As a general rule, then, cold is a tonic to the skin, and heat debilitates it."[9]

Bathing for personal cleanliness was, perhaps, more controversial than "taking the waters" to prevent or cure illness. In the nineteenth century, spas located in the vicinity of natural springs were popular resorts for health and recreation. Indeed, McLean County boasted its own such facility, Sulfur Springs near Carlock, which during the late nineteenth century had a hotel and several cottages to which vacationers and health seekers flocked. Hydropathy was used, both to cure and to strengthen. As we have seen, Dr. Henry Conkling of Bloomington opened his Turkish and Electro-Thermal Institute in 1870, providing a local alternative to heroic cures. Catharine Beecher was also an advocate of Water Cures, calling them "the safest and surest methods of relieving debilitated constitutions and curing chronic ailments." She maintained that water treatments, which involved internal and external applications of cold water, were more effective and safer than commonly used medicines, writing, "After these processes have been fairly tried, few would ever wish to return to medicines as a remedy for . . . most common ailments."[10]

Nonetheless, there was no general consensus that bathing was necessary to either health or beauty. Neither bodies nor clothes were frequently washed. In an age before mass production of cheap and easily accessible cotton clothing, many garments did not wash well. It is, perhaps, not surprising that, except among the prosperous classes, sensibilities were not as refined as they later became. Body odor was accepted and unremarked.

Contemporary concern about diseases of filth (mainly typhus, typhoid and cholera) were associated not with personal but with environmental dirt.

Human Waste

. . . We had our posy garden that the women loved so well,
   I loved it too, but better still I loved the stronger smell
   That filled the evening breezes so full of homely cheer,
   And told the night-o'ertaken tramp that human life was near.
   On lazy August afternoons, it made a little bower
   Delightful, where my grandsire sat and whiled away an hour.
   For there the summer mornings its very cares entwined,
   And berry bushes reddened in the steaming soil behind.

   . . . When Grandpa had to "go out back" and make his morning call,
   We'd bundle up the dear old man with a muffler and a shawl,
   I knew the hole on which he sat, 'twas padded all around
   And once I dared to sit there — 'twas all too wide I found,
   My loins were all too little and I jack-knifed there to stay,
   They had to come and get me out or I'd have passed away.
   Then Father said ambition was a thing that boys should shun,
   And I just use the children's hole 'til childhood days were done.

   And still I marvel at the craft that cut those holes so true,
   The baby hole, and the slender hole that fitted Sister Sue.
   That dear old country landmark; I've tramped around a bit,
   And in the lap of luxury my lot has been to sit —
   But e'er I die I'll eat the fruit of trees I robbed of yore
   Then seek the shanty where my name is carved upon the door,
   I ween the old familiar smell will soothe my faded soul,
   I'm now a man, but none the less I'll try the children's hole.

"Passing of the Back-House" attributed to James Whitcomb Riley[11]

Traditionally, people were more concerned about keeping their bowels open than about where their feces went. Though less deadly than diarrhea, constipation was more widely feared because it was generally thought to herald virtually all kinds of illness. Retention of waste was believed to poison the whole system. Both curative and preventative medicine, therefore, advised regular use of laxatives and enemas to keep the bowels clean and the body "soluble." Health experts agreed that virtually all aspects of hygiene should focus on producing regularity. They had nothing to say, however, about healthy methods of waste disposal, because until the late nineteenth century there was only one available means — the outdoor privy.

Except in cities, where crowded buildings meant that privies were attached to housing and waste was either carried away or thrown into open sewers, it was customary to locate outhouses "out back", at some distance from homes and other buildings. When one pit filled up, another location on the property could be chosen and the outhouse moved. "Wells were always uphill (if possible) and a safe distance away from the privy, and were generally more convenient to the house."[12] As towns became more crowded, available space for outhouses became increasingly limited and pollution of water sources inevitable. McLean County, located on flat, low land, was particularly vulnerable to water-borne illnesses such as typhoid, which increased in incidence during the second half of the nineteenth century. According to an article published in a Bloomington newspaper, *The Pantagraph*, in 1875:

> The local order is to usually locate your house in front, the well in the rear of the house, and the stables, pig pens, privies, etc. in the rear of the well. Often the privies and wells are higher than the house for access to the street. Such results in a chronically damp cellar from the stable and privy fluids. The distance between well and privy is generally 30 feet. The instances are very numerous in which the poison of typhoid fever has been traced to water that had traversed the soil many feet . . . . In view of the way porous soil extends in this city . . . are we not compelled to infer- ence that our wells are impure and unsafe. The wells of the city are so open and unprotected that any amount of sur- face drainage and filth may enter them.[13]

The first American patent for a flush toilet was awarded in 1833, and by the 1850s many upper- and middle-class houses in eastern cities had installed them.[14] However, McLean County was slow to follow this trend. "Clover Lawn," the mansion built by David and Sarah Davis in Bloomington in 1872, was apparently the first home in the county to have a flush toilet.[15] Since the city's sewer system was not developed until the 1880s, the Davis's plumbing probably emptied into a septic system or cesspool.[16]

Even in the twentieth century, when indoor toilets were routinely installed in towns, some householders continued to maintain backyard facilities for servants, guests and others who did not trust these new-fangled gadgets. Rural residents had fewer health reasons for and greater financial objections to installation of flush toilets. Thus, particularly in rural areas, outhouses remained common in McLean County until after World War II.

Public Health in McLean County

The Fight Against Contagion

Informal public health activities are as old as the county. The chief concern was to prevent the introduction of diseases known to be contagious into settled communities. Newcomers were regarded with suspicion. This study has already referred to the eagerness of early residents of Blooming Grove to exile from the community a mother and child suffering from smallpox.[17] As the population grew and travel became easier (largely due to the development of railway networks), communities implemented more formal means of dealing with the threat of epidemic illness. After about 1870, in years when diseases such as smallpox, yellow fever and cholera were known to be epidemic elsewhere in the region, it was not uncommon for Bloomington officials to forbid passengers to disembark from trains coming from the direction of infected areas.[18] A local smallpox outbreak in Shirley in the mid-1870s stimulated both the quarantine of the entire township and vaccination of all school children.[19]

In order to isolate cases, in 1878 a house isolated on the outskirts of Bloomington was adopted as a "pesthouse".[20] This was used for people who could not be quarantined in their own homes. According to reports regarding the 1882 smallpox epidemic,

> Tramps, immigrants and new-comers came under the ban of epidemiological scrutiny at this time and, as usually happened, local officials pinned the blame of starting the epidemic upon a couple of tramps, an immigrant and a family of new-comers who happened to be still within the limits of the honeymoon period of their matrimonial experience. The bride and groom escaped the "pesthouse" because of their advanced convalescence, but the unhappy vagabonds paid for their indiscretion by a solitary residence in that isolated institution. . . .[21]

More usual than institutional confinement, however, was for sufferers to be quarantined in their own homes. As an increasing number of diseases were identified as communicable after 1880, home quarantine became both customary and legally imposed. The front doors of the homes of sufferers were sign-posted, and residents who could not be absent from work often lived away from home. A release for the convalescent patient from the attending physician became necessary before ordinary contact with the community was thought to be safe. Thus, in 1907, the McLean County Medical Society was asked to advise a local school board about the proper length of time a child who had had an infectious disease should be kept home from school (two weeks).[22] After the patient had recovered, sickrooms, equipment, bed linen and clothing were fumigated. In 1898, 18 cases of scarlet fever and 15 cases of diphtheria were recorded for Bloomington, "with a notation that all cases had been quarantined and the premises fumigated after termination of the illness."[23] Until after World War II, sufferers from diphtheria, measles, scarlet fever, whooping cough and mumps, together with other members of their households, were quarantined in their homes.

Sanitation and Public Services

More significant than attempts to prevent or limit the spread of contagious diseases, however, were development of formal sanitation policies and public services. These depended upon population growth and local perceptions of need. Such policies and services were implemented earlier in large eastern cities than in the smaller new communities of the west. However, as these communities grew, they got dirty. First publicized by the British sanitarian Sir Edwin Chadwick and American activists such as Boston's Lemuel Shattuck and John Griscom of New York, the relationship between dirt and disease was well established. Both individuals and communities were encouraged by such reformers to clean up their environments.

In McLean County, as elsewhere, public sanitation activities began in urban areas. An initial step in collective hygiene was to rid streets of livestock. According to one authority:

> Prior to April of 1871 when an ordinance was passed restraining people from letting livestock run at large, roving herds of pigs, chickens, goats, and an occasional cow ran wild through the streets of Bloomington. These ani-

mals did probably provide the city with a valuable service, the first street cleaning, but in their wake left piles of waste, which was likely not often cleaned from the predominantly mud streets.[24]

Unpaved surfaces were difficult to clean. Thus, paving was an important public health measure. Paving of Bloomington's streets began in 1869 with the laying of crushed gravel on a stretch of Grove Street. Several other streets were paved with wood blocks, which were abandoned in favor of brick pavement beginning in 1877.[25] The streets of Normal, and other communities in the County, were not paved until after the turn of the century.

More important to health than general clean-up was the development of public water supplies. Only Philadelphia, New York and Boston had public waterworks before the 1860s. The lack of a large natural water source was a matter of concern to McLean County from the earliest years of settlement. According to one historian:

> The dry year of 1854 caused great distress for water in this part of the State, and Bloomington people were very much exercised with fears that the location and building of their rapidly-growing city might, after all, have been a serious mistake. . . . A public meeting was called July 23, 1854, when Mr. J.W. Fell offered . . . resolutions which were unanimously adopted after a discussion, in which the mover, Judge Davis, Dr. Freese and others participated.[26]

Resolutions included organizing a committee including members with engineering expertise to create plans for development of a public water supply. In the attempt to find a local coal supply, Bloomington had sunk a coal shaft in 1863. Although no coal was found, the drill struck an underground water source, which in 1869 was tapped by the Chicago and Alton Railroad Company for its own uses. This success stimulated the city to solve its water problems by digging a well — an initiative undertaken in 1874 "at the end of a series of four very dry seasons": [27]

> On Christmas Day, 1874, the whole population that wished, examined the fountain — the well having been finished the day before. As a sample of what had been discovered, the engines were kept at work, throwing the water in a stream which, as it flowed off, was equal to a good-sized brook.

There was but one opinion, and that was that the fountain was large enough to justify the erection of a system of water works; and in the summer of 1875, the stand-pipe was erected, 200 feet high, an engine and pump placed in position at the well, two miles and a half of pipe laid in the streets, and a full system of water works inaugurated, which has since been enlarged by additional pipes and more machinery. The total cost of the whole, up to April 30, 1878, has been $86,944.83. This includes about eight miles of water-mains, the engines and machinery, the stand-pipe, four drinking fountains, seventy hydrants and everything connected with the Water Department.[28]

Although this development was generally celebrated, many home-owners were unwilling to install the expensive new plumbing necessary to connect their houses with the public water supply. Indeed, in August, 1878, only 50 families drew water from the city well, while 3,000 continued to use private wells.[29] Only approximately 85 percent of homes were using city water in 1925.[30] Thus, acceptance of public services was gradual, and tended to be associated with new construction.

While the first public well provided a temporary solution to Bloomington's water problems, population growth and occasional dry seasons pressured the city to expand its water works several times (1885, 1909). Both quantity and quality of the city's water supply continued to be subjects of general concern, stimulating development in the 1920s of a citizen's committee charged with studying alternatives for establishment of a suitable water supply.[31] In 1929, an earth dam 45 feet high and 800 feet long was built on Money Creek, creating Lake Bloomington, which is located about 14 miles away from the city. A water treatment plant was constructed in 1933, after which time Bloomington's old wells were abandoned. The city's water supply was augmented in 1972 by the completion of Evergreen Lake.[32]

At the same time Bloomington was developing its public water supply, its citizens were directing their attention to the question of public management of waste water and sewage. Before the 1870s, all kinds of garbage and human and animal waste had been thrown into what became know as the "North and South Sloughs," originally small streams running into Sugar Creek. Over the years, the Sloughs " became a . . . sodden pool of stench that was the breeding place for disease . . . because it drained sewage into the community's primary water source, Sugar

Creek."[33] The nuisance and health risk became so great that in 1874 construction on a new sewerage system began:

> The unsightly holes of the North and South Sloughs were covered by large tile pipes that carried the sewage underground away from the city. . . . Hotel builders and private landowners paid the cost of their own installation. Other buildings were drained through plank or box sewers which were installed from year to year. The box sewers were square wooden ducts running underground from a business or residence to a larger box collecting drain.[34]

These sewers were built to drain north and westward into Sugar Creek, "there being in 1920 seven such sewers ranging from 15 to 96 inches in diameter."[35]

As with public water service, residents were slow about becoming connected to the sewerage system. Outhouses were cheaper, and people were accustomed to using them. Indeed, some felt that it was more hygienic for people to void their waste outside of their homes than in them. Thus, in 1925, it was estimated that only 80 percent of Bloomington's dwellings were connected with sewers.[36]

During its first fifty years of operation, the sewerage system continued to dump untreated waste into Sugar Creek. However, in the late 1920s, a sewage treatment plant was built to serve the newly organized Bloomington-Normal Sanitary District. This development resulted from two law suits filed in 1919 on behalf of rural landowners against the City of Bloomington, Town of Normal, and several factories located along Sugar Creek. Alex Bryant, one of the plaintiffs, was a farmer residing northwest of Bloomington who protested the pollution of the stream which crossed his property. "Mr. Bryant represented that the water which flowed over his farm for quite a distance so poisoned the crops that they were unfit to feed the stock and that the water created an unsanitary condition about his premises causing he [sic] and his family to become ill." In 1925, the case was decided in favor of the plaintiffs. Bloomington and Normal were ordered to clean up the mess and begin to implement plans for the sewage treatment facility which began operations in 1928.[37]

Public Health Administration

The Illinois State Board of Health was established in 1877 to administer two laws: the Medical Practice Act, which regulated the professional practice of medicine, and the State Board of Health Act, which administered sanitation, quarantines and collection of health statistics in the state. This development was, in part, spearheaded by Dr. E.W. Gray of Bloomington, who in 1876 had delivered a paper on the sanitary control of disease for the annual meeting of the Illinois State Medical Society.[38]

Bloomington had been at the forefront of public health developments, having established its City Health Board in 1842.[39] Becoming more active in such matters as time went on, by 1880 the City Council had established a Health Committee which employed a Health Officer, Hiram Greenwood, for $40.00 per month. His responsibilities included:

> abatement of nuisances and the enforcement of garbage removal regulations. He had police powers and . . . was responsible for removing to the "pesthouse" persons found in the community with smallpox.[40]

Greenwood held his position until 1898.

While local physicians were not initially officially associated with the Committee, the McLean County Medical Society was extremely interested both in its activities and in the sanitary conditions prevailing in the city of Bloomington. For example, the Society's records indicate that in 1891 members were offended by a city regulation requiring them to report cases of diphtheria to the Health Officer, and allowing that official to visit sufferers in the absence of their own doctors. This tension between physicians and public health personnel reflects national trends. While advocating state regulation of medical practice, organized medicine resented public infringement on private practice and public provision of health care.[41] Bloomington's physicians opted to control local health administration, rather than fight with it. Concerned about local sanitary conditions, in 1897 the Medical Society organized a committee to advocate appointment of a physician as Medical Officer.[42] This committee was successful in its activities, securing a part-time appointment of Dwight O. Moore, M.D., in 1898. Serving under Moore was a Sanitary Policeman, John F. Anderson, who presumably undertook the nuisance abatement and enforcement activities previously performed by Greenwood. Thereafter, the Medical Society and the Bloomington Health Committee generally worked amicably together.

The Health Committee performed an increasing range of functions as time went on. After 1901, the Health Commissioner began to keep vital statistics for the city. Previously, these figures had been kept by the county clerk. Then, after 1915, under the supervision of between one and three local physicians, the Commission for Public Health and Safety employed two inspectors; one for foods and one for sanitation. Also during the first decades of the century, a small laboratory was established to run tests on food and milk and for certain diseases (diphtheria and gonorrhea in particular). Other types of tests were conducted in Springfield. Nurses began to be employed by the Commission early in the twentieth century, particularly to support the health of infants, school children and tuberculosis patients. These nurses made home and school visits, conducted a day nursery and promoted health education and hygiene through local mothers' clubs. In 1921, Dr. J.M. Furstman became one of the first full-time Health Commissioners to be employed in Illinois outside of Chicago. He was assisted by three nurses and two inspectors. [43]

This administrative structure served Bloomington for some years, with people from outlying areas taking advantage of certain services, including the Fairview Tuberculosis Sanitorium. Also promoting public health activities, particularly in the rural areas, was the county's first Home Bureau advisor, Clara Brian, who began work in 1918. Brian was active in health education, promoting healthy cooking and diet, school meals programs and fly eradication. In addition, she was instrumental in the establishment of the McLean County Health Department in 1945.[44]

This department routinized inspection, immunization, health education and vision and hearing screening services. In addition, it administered a growing range of public health services provided to the poor and elderly. As Ben Boyd, who began working as a sanitarian in Illinois in 1955 and became the Director of Environmental Health in McLean County in 1966, said, "The physicians get narrowed in on their individual patients and they don't think about the community as a patient. Of course, that's our [public health workers'] focus. The community is our patient, not the individual."[45]

Battling Tuberculosis

Tuberculosis was the leading cause of death in McLean County before the twentieth century, "ordinarily accounting for more fatalities than any other disease."[46] Before Koch's discovery of the tubercle bacillus in 1882, the disease was not commonly regarded as contagious. Thus, while individual attempts were made to prevent tuberculosis by cultivating a generally healthy lifestyle, and a wide range of therapies was applied once the disease had appeared, no collective approaches to either prevention or cure were devised. Diagnosis of tuberculosis, which was often delayed because there were no conclusive tests available, was commonly regarded as a death sentence.

This situation changed around the turn of the century, as the various means of transmission of pulmonary and other types of tuberculosis were identified. Prevention activities included anti-spitting ordinances, prohibition of the sale of milk from tuberculous cattle and attempts to isolate the sick from the well. Many communities began systematically to collect case and contact reports in order to track and treat the tuberculous.[47] Anti-tuberculosis activists also developed sites for administration of the open-air cure, which was thought to be the best treatment for consumptives. In 1906 the Chicago Tuberculosis Institute established an open-air camp for poor sufferers living in congested areas of the city, while the Illinois Homeopathic Medical Association founded an open-air sanitarium at Buffalo Rock in LaSalle County.[48]

Bloomington's medical community was very concerned about tuberculosis. Interest had been stimulated at the 1904 annual meeting of the Illinois State Medical Society, which convened in Bloomington. In March of 1907, the McLean County Medical Society called a public meeting, which was addressed by Dr. J.W. Pettit of the Ottawa Tent Colony. He argued that tuberculosis was:

> only feebly contagious under certain conditions which can easily be avoided — i.e., by destruction of all sputa. The uncontrolled patient only is a menace. Sanitoria, properly conducted, are the safest places possible because of control had over the patient. Physicians and nurses at sanitoria are practically free from disease. The great work of sanitoria is in what they teach the patient, and through him the public, towards limiting the spread of disease.[49]

Concerned citizens formed an organization later named the McLean County Anti-tuberculosis Society to support enactment of a state law permitting counties to levy a tax to maintain sanitoria. Such a law, named "Glackin" after the state senator who proposed it, was passed in 1908.

McLean County was among the first in the state to take advantage of this law, passing a referendum in 1916 to establish a sanitarium. This facility, which would be known as Fairview, opened in August 1919. Meanwhile, the Anti-tuberculosis Society hired a visiting nurse and carried on extensive educational work among families which included sufferers.

Fairview Sanitarium was built on a pleasant rise north of Normal at a cost of $125,000. Initially able to care for 34 patients at a time, it was enlarged to accommodate a total of 49 within the main building. During the 1920s, "three new rooms, six beds and a cottage for colored people" were added.[50] Care, which often lasted for years, was free to McLean County residents. In addition to the sanitarium, a free public dispensary serving TB sufferers was opened in 1918 in downtown Bloomington. Medical director Dr. Bernice Curry, who also served as director of the Fairview Sanitarium, and the nurse, Mrs. Brett, saw 333 cases in 1918 alone.

Mortality from tuberculosis declined dramatically after the introduction of streptomycin in the late 1940s. Nonetheless, Fairview Sanitarium was supported by county tax funds until 1965, when the facility closed due to lack of patients.[51] After this time, residents of the county suffering from tuberculosis received tax support for care in other institutions in the state. The building was later adapted for use by the McLean County Health Department.

Conclusions

Our culture has been profoundly influenced by the parallel activities of biomedical researchers, sanitation engineers, health policy advocates and health educators. We wash our hands after using flush toilets, consume food and drugs marketed under strict governmental regulations, and clean household surfaces with powerful chemicals known to "kill germs" because of their efforts. Virtually all of our physical activities, from tooth-care to sex, are informed by conventional wisdom about healthy (and unhealthy) ways to do things. Our increasing longevity and health in old age testify to the fact that an ounce of prevention is indeed worth a pound of cure.

Yet, compared to medical therapeutics, public health and hygiene have tended to assume the position of the poor relation or ugly sister. Transplant surgery makes headlines, while health education can barely find space in school curricula. Our society still struggles with the question of whether to devote more resources to preventing or to curing disease. Yet, experts agree that prevention promises the most cost effective and humane solution to modern health problems.[52] Especially in an era when chronic diseases, whether infectious or not, have become the major killers, public policies and dollars supporting healthy environments and lifestyles will be well spent.

Health in a Bottle: Patent Medicines and Self-Treatment

The Development of the Trade

The sale of patent medicines in North America began before the American Revolution. In general, these nostrums came into being in someone's kitchen or resulted from chemical or distilling experiments. Thus, the distinction between home remedies and patent medicines is often blurred. However, the main difference is that patent, or proprietary, remedies are, in theory at least, compounded from the same recipe each time they are made, packaged and sold to a market extending beyond the maker's household or neighborhood. The concept of a patent medicine dates back to sixteenth-century England, when "patents were monopolies granted at the pleasure of the soveriegn, to encourage various skills and manufactures."[1]

Many "patent" remedies were never patented at all. According to one authority on the American nostrum industry:

> Proprietors who chose to patent their formulas boasted that this step signified governmental endorsement of therapeutic efficacy. In exchange for the . . . right to make this . . . claim, those securing patents had to reveal each medicine's composition. Most proprietors preferred to vend secret formulas without a patent. The term "patent medicine" came in common parlance to apply to both categories indistinguishably.[2]

Since the exclusive right to vend a patented compound legally ended seventeen years after the patent was issued, most vendors chose to patent, not their recipes, but the manufacturer's trademark.[3]

In traditional Europe, it was usual for both official and irregular medical practitioners to develop their own, often "secret", remedies for sale, either as part of supervised treatment or to be used as the purchaser chose.[4] Exclusive knowledge of the composition of these medicines added to the practitioner's market appeal. Many of them contained exotic ingredients, such as "unicorn's horn", "mummy" or gold. There was also a fashion in sixteenth- and seventeenth-century England for the medicinal use of ingredients obtained in newly discovered parts of the globe. Coffee, tea, chocolate and tobacco were used for their supposed healing properties, while substances such as opium and "Jesuit's bark" (containing the effective agent found in quinine) gained apparently permanent places in the Western pharmacopoeia. This period also witnessed the development of "Paracelsian", or non-herbal, remedies, which contained ingredients such as mercury, arsenic, antimony and lead.[5]

The more complicated the recipe, the greater the claims made for it by the doctor or apothecary who sold it. Some compounds promised a specific effect, which was usually purgative. More common were the tonics, which offered a general pick-me-up, and panaceas, which cured everything from nasal congestion to cancer. The doctors, apothecaries and quacks who became involved in the over-the-counter medicine trade in nineteenth-century America thus inherited a long tradition. However, the trade blossomed during that period as a result of new circumstances, including industrialization, western expansion and technological developments.

While, in the early years of the century, Americans imported from Europe most of the prepared medications and medical instruments they needed:

> From the 1820s and 1830s onward. . . small native laboratories, many of them in Philadelphia, began producing a variety of chemicals, patent medicines, and other preparations. Similarly, in small shops, American artisans designed and began the production of a growing range of surgical, dental, and other instruments and equipment.[6]

The production, marketing and distribution of prepared remedies was greatly enhanced in mid-century by development of industrial production methods; improved transportation and postal systems; and proliferation of advertising vehicles. These innovations met the challenge of an increasingly dispersed population, which depended upon often distant urban centers to fill their need for manufactured goods of all kinds.

Nostrum factories sprang up all over the country. By the 1850s, Midwesterners did not have to rely upon eastern suppliers, but could purchase mass produced, mass marketed remedies much closer to home. An active mail-order trade also flourished, supported by newspaper, leaflet and almanac advertisements; traveling salesmen; and catalogues. This trade was stimulated by expansion of a national railroad network, affording both middlemen and consumers access to an enormous range of both homegrown and foreign patent medicines. The foreign and exotic continued to have a marketing edge. In the 1850s McLean County newspapers advertised Dr. John Bull's Sarsaparilla, German Liniment and Dr. Morse's Indian Root Pills.

This nostrum trade was entirely unregulated, and benefited both from the heroic dosing common among regular physicians and from the significant opposition to heroic remedies among alternative practitioners and sufferers. Consumers purchased the powerful laxatives and emetics they thought necessary to "clean themselves out"; they also bought "painless, nice-tasting, and non-mineral . . . proprietary products" marketed as superior to the allopaths' mercury and jalap.[7]

Who supplied these remedies? The term "patent medicine" has long been associated with its popular equivalent, "snake oil."[8] Cures marketed by itinerant quacks and advertisements in the popular press lured the ignorant, unwary and desperate with promises the orthodox healers of the period could not make. (They also invariably sought respectability by warning readers to beware of the dangerous charlatans who threatened both their purses and their lives.) Patent remedies offered relief from incurable miseries such as consumption, cancer, epilepsy and insanity. They catered to concern about "new" diseases such as neurasthenia, the debility affecting many middle-class women, and the "disease of masturbation." They also filled family medicine chests for use in everyday ailments such as headaches, constipation, stomach complaints and fevers. Composed of ingredients ranging from herbs and roots, to those of mineral and animal origin, they often also included alcohol, opiates and cocaine.

Patent medicines were sold during performances of traveling medicine shows, where consumers received both entertainment and hope of relief for the price of a bottle. Bloomington annually hosted a number of these troops, which in the 1880s included Bigelow's Kickapoo Indian Shows and Healey's Kickapoo Indian Shows.[9]

Nostrum-makers also advertised in newspapers, pouring as much as 50 percent of their profits back into advertising.[10] Virtually every town had at least one daily or weekly paper, and every paper advertised patent medicines. Advertisements provided both information about the remedy and testimonials about its efficacy. For example, Donald Kennedy of Roxbury, Massachusetts, advertised "The Greatest Medical Discovery of the Age," which was based upon "one of our common pasture weeds" (never identified). According to its publicist:

> Nothing looks so improbable to those who have in vain tried all the wonderful medicines of the day, as that a common weed growing on the pastures and along solid stone walls should cure every humor in the system, yet it is a fixed fact. . . . I peddled over a thousand bottles of it in the vicinity of Boston — I know the effects of it in every case. It has already done some of the greatest cures ever done in Massachusetts. I gave it children a year old, to old people of sixty. I have seen poor, puny, wormy-looking children, whose flesh was soft and flabby, restored to a perfect state of health by one bottle. To those who are subject to a sick head ache, one bottle will always cure it. It gives great relief in catarrh and dizziness. Some who have taken it have been costive [i.e., constipated] for years, and have been regulated by it. Where the body is sound it works easy, but where there is any derangement of the functions of nature, it will cause very singular feelings, but you must not be alarmed: they always disappear in from four to six weeks.[11]

Like many other remedies, this one sold for $1 a bottle. While by today's standards this price was comparatively inexpensive, by those of the 1850s, it was a significant expenditure. Further, most ailments required more than one bottle. Two bottles were "warranted to cure a nursing sore mouth" (possibly scurvy), three to five bottles were needed for "the worst kind of erysipelas" (also called St. Anthony's Fire), and five to eight bottles cured scrofula. Along with other proprietary remedies, this one was distributed by drug stores as well as by mail order. In Bloomington it was sold by no fewer than four retail firms.

In addition to being sold by mail and over the counter, patent medicines were sold by regular physicians. Indeed, most doctors sold drugs, and many owned and operated drug stores. For example, Dr. Stevenson, who arrived in Chenoa in 1857, operated a drug store in the town for some years.[12] Dr. Rogers, who practiced in Bloomington in the 1850s prescribed and sold proprietary remedies out of his office.[13] In 1879, Dr. Waters of Lexington had his office at the People's Drug Store, which he also operated; Dr. H. Parkhurst of Danvers was also proprietor of the City Drug Store; and Dr. Samuel D. Wright of Stanford billed himself in a county directory as "physician, surgeon and druggist."[14]

Some large drug companies saw the advantage of utilizing physicians as the chief salesmen for their products, selling so-called "ethical" drugs mainly by prescription even before the drug trade was officially regulated.[15] In 1899 the Bayer company of Germany introduced its new preparation, aspirin, as an ethical drug, and did not advertise it as an over-the-counter medicine until the second decade of the twentieth century. Patients became familiar with the medicine upon a physician's recommendation, purchasing it directly from druggists thereafter. For example,

> As late as 1915, Fellow's Proprietary Syrup was still being promoted exclusively to physicians, with not one cent spent on direct advertising to the consumer, but 90 percent of its sales were over-the-counter without a doctor's prescription.[16]

Then as now, physicians' recommendations were linked to self-medication and sales of proprietary remedies. Aspirin provides a useful example because, together with other non-prescription pain-relievers, it remains a staple for both official therapy and self-medication. Even in the late twentieth century, when both the cultural authority of physicians and popular expectations of professional medicine are far greater than they had been a century before, people continue to dose themselves for a wide range of minor and chronic health problems. Headaches, arthritis, indigestion, menstrual cramps, sinus congestion, constipation and a host of other discomforts still tend to be treated at home before they are taken to the doctor.

The Promise of Cure

In the nineteenth century, despite their efforts and hopes, people did not *expect* their illnesses to be cured. However, they did expect the medicine they took to relieve certain symptoms and became familiar with the effects of a multitude of remedies, which they often used instead of consulting physicians. Laxatives and emetics, often combined with enemas, relieved constipation. The alcohol base of many nostrums made some sufferers feel better, regardless of their efficacy against the disease causing the symptoms. Syrups such as "Grandma's Secret," "Mother's Treasure" and "Mrs. Winslow's Soothing Syrup," which were laced with opium, morphine and cocaine, relieved pain and soothed (and sometimes killed) fretful babies.[17] In addition to medicines which were expected to "work," in the sense of having a specific effect, people took tonics which they believed strengthened them and helped to prevent illness. Thus, generations of children grew up with Scott's Emulsion of Cod Liver Oil, which was also thought to be particularly good for tuberculosis sufferers.

The sales pitches for patent medicines were based upon accepted medical theories. Mr. Kennedy's cure-all, referred to above, promised to "cure every humor in the system." This rather garbled promise indicates both the longevity of humoralism and the developing view of human bodies as complicated physiological systems which operated predictably and similarly. Following contemporary ideas about the origin of fevers, an 1850s advertisement for an ague remedy admonished the reader,

> Tonics won't do! They never did do more than give temporary relief and they never will. It is because they don't touch the CAUSE of the disease — The cause of all ague and bilious diseases is the atmospheric poison called Miasma or Malaria. Neutralize this poison by its Natural Antidote and all diseases caused by it disappears at once. Rhodes' Fever and Ague cure is Antidote to Malaria, and moreover it is a perfectly harmless medicine . . . .
> Therefore, if it does no good, it can do no harm.[18]

While nostrums were available for all kinds of ailments, certain categories of sufferers were especially targeted by patent medicine manufacturers. People suffering from disorders they considered to be shameful, such as sexually transmitted diseases, impotence or addiction, received special attention. For example, Dr. Baker's Specific was billed as "a safe and certain cure for gonorrhea, gleet, stricture, seminal weakness, and all diseases of the genital organs":

> It is very agreeable to the taste, creates no perceptible odor, and may be used . . . with entire secrecy, without regard to diet, hindrance from business or medical advisor, as plain directions for use accompany the medicine. Reader, have you private disease? Do not neglect it. Delay is dangerous![19]

One Chicago mail-order doctor offered, instead of medication, a "treatise" which he promised would cure young men of the "special disease of Masturbation," writing:

> The following disorders, some in one case, some in another,

are again the direct consequences of this disease, *viz.*:
Seminal Emissions, General Debility and Nervousness,
Distaste for Society, Gloomy Presentments, weakness in the
back, impairment of . . . memory, weak and watery eyes,
eruptions on skin and body, restlessness or vicious dreams.
. . unfitness for marriage relationships, excitability of the
organs, strictures, costiveness, dyspepsia, etc.[20]

The volume of advertisements indicate that alcoholism and
addiction to opiates (mainly opium and morphine) were viewed as
increasing problems as the nineteenth century progressed. This
perception may be related to the development of the temperance
movement during the same period. It is also related to both physicians' routine prescription of remedies containing alcohol and opiates and to sufferers' routine resort to over-the-counter medications containing the same ingredients. Whatever the reason, the
problem was perceived to be a largely male one, and the audience
targeted by advertisements was female — generally, the long-suf-
fering wife. Thus, the January 1900 issue of *The People's Home
Journal* contained an advertisement entitled "Drink Habit Cured."
It went on to say:

Any true woman might well be proud to have saved one
poor soul from the shackles of drink, but Mrs. Hawkins has
redeemed thousands by her noble and practical work
among those who have been victims of intemperance. Mrs.
Hawkins for years suffered the grief and anguish shared
by so many true and faithful women of America today, who
have drink-afflicted fathers, husbands or sons. She determined to overcome this fearful evil if possible. Her search
for a harmless, perfect and secret home cure was at last
rewarded when an old friend came to her and gave her a
remedy which had never been known to fail. Mrs. Hawkins
gave the remedy secretly and in a few weeks, to her great
joy, her dearest relative was entirely cured of his appetite
for drink and was again restored to health and man-
hood. . . . With the assistance of others she perfected the
original treatment and now offers to send this treatment
free to any distressed wife, mother or sister who will write
for it.[21]

Mrs. Hawkins was unusually generous, but it is probable that, as
was the case for other preparations, only the trial treatment was
free. Like cures for morphine, laudanum, opium and tobacco
addiction, this remedy was to be placed secretly in the addict's cof-

fee or tea by the concerned wife, sister or mother. Treatment was supposed to be painless, and the "patient" cured without his own knowledge. However, these cures often lasted a very long time because the medicines usually contained opiates in a concealed form.[22]

Advertisements for patent remedies serve as an early source for a phenomenon which has received more attention in the twentieth century: iatrogenic illness (i.e., illness caused by medical treatment). Addiction to opium, morphine, laudanum, cocaine and codeine was very likely to have a medical origin, since so many remedies, whether prescribed by a physician or self-administered, contained these ingredients. Indeed, so common was addiction to narcotics following treatment of old war wounds that it was known as the "army disease."[23]

Also common were the symptoms of mercury poisoning which resulted from ingestion of calomel — a mercury derivative which was taken as routinely as late-twentieth-century sufferers take Tylenol. A poem, published in 1910 when the remedy had gone out of fashion, probably drew an accurate picture of earlier dosing practices:

> When Mr. A. or B. is sick
> Go call the doctor, and be quick.
> The doctor comes with much good will,
> And gives a case of Calomel.
>
> He takes the patient by the hand
> And compliments him as a friend.
> He sits awhile his pulse to feel,
> And then takes out his Calomel.
>
> He then turns to the patient's wife,
> "Have you clean paper, spoon and knife?
> I think your husband would do well
> To take a dose of Calomel."
>
> He then deals out the precious grain.
> "This, ma'am, I'm sure will ease the pain.
> Once in three hours at toll of bell
> Give him a dose of Calomel."
>
> The man grows worse, quite fast indeed.
> "Go call the doctor, ride with speed."
> The doctor comes like post with mail

Doubling his dose of Calomel.

The man in death begins to groan.
The fatal job for him is done.
He dies, alas, but sure to tell,
A sacrifice to Calomel.

And when I must resign my breath,
Pray let me die a natural death
And bid the world a long farewell,
Without a dose of Calomel.[24]

Nostrum-makers identified mercury poisoning as an ailment caused by regular physicians, and particularly appropriate for their attention. An advertisement for Dr. Easterly's Iodine and Sarsaparilla, promised that the medicine cured most diseases by "driving out and radically removing all diseased and impure fluids from the body." Further, "it is the only safe and sure remedy for thoroughly eradicating mercury from the system and for the cure of secondary syphilis and venereal diseases." Since mercury was routinely prescribed for syphilis, this remedy promised to cure the sufferer of both the disease and the treatment.[25]

Another market especially targeted by nostrum-makers was women. Disorders associated with the female reproductive system were especially problematical in the nineteenth century. Culture, environment and medical theory and practice combined both to cause and to popularize conditions such as neurasthenia (general debility and nervousness thought to be the result of disordered female reproductive organs), uterine displacement and prolapse, and malfunction of the ovaries. Women's clothing, which constricted the mid-section and suspended the heavy weight of skirts and undergarments from the waist, was blamed for all of these conditions. Middle-class women's sedentary lifestyles were also thought to be unhealthy. Further, damage resulting from childbearing — particularly from instrument-aided intervention by surgeons — resulted in conditions such as prolapse and incontinence, which made invalids of many women.[26]

Until the nineteenth century "female problems" had been an exclusively female province, treated, if at all, by midwives and amateur healers. Despite the fact that male physicians and surgeons became increasingly interested in the developing fields of obstetrics and gynecology in the 1800s, escalating female modesty militated against women consulting male practitioners except in extreme cases.[27] Modesty, shame and fear of public exposure were particularly important for female sufferers from venereal diseases.

In addition, women had reason to be concerned about the trend, supported by the twin developments of anesthetics and antiseptic surgical procedures, in favor of using surgery to solve a range of ailments identified as "female problems," including moodiness, weakness and inappropriate sexual behavior, in addition to ovarian and uterine tumors and the variety of structural problems which were complications of childbirth injuries.[28] This trend was the subject of a discussion which occurred at a regular meeting of the McLean County Medical Society in July, 1897, during which Dr. John L. White maintained that "many needless ovariotomies were performed and that, in general, for the various neuroses of women, surgery was a failure."[29]

Virtually all symptoms suffered by women were interpreted on the basis of their reproductive organs. Modest women would do much to avoid the internal examination necessary for diagnosis. Furthermore, the treatments prescribed by doctors, including surgery, application of strong chemicals or cautery to the vagina, or the use of pessaries to keep the errant womb in its place, tended to be both embarrassing and painful. Thus, women turned to patent remedies before consulting physicians. A wide range of nostrums promised everything from beautiful skin to relief from venereal disease. Thus, Dr. Hooper's Female Cordial was marketed in the 1850s as:

> A safe and sure remedy for Female Complaints arising
> from debility, such as Irregularity or Suppression of the
> Menses, Fluer Albus or Whites, Barrenness, Sallow
> Complexion, Headache, Dizziness, Weak Nerves, Frightful
> Dreams, and all diseases caused by Colds, Checked
> Perspiration, Excesses, over-excitement, etc.[30]

The anonymity of the mail-order medicine trade also offered women a greater degree of control over their fertility than local doctors did. In an age when contraception was not discussed and abortion was shameful, dangerous and illegal, distant nostrum sellers offered one alternative to the unmarried girls fearing public shame or mothers of many who were unwilling to face the prospect of another mouth to feed. Many of the remedies sold to women contained the implied promise that they would keep the menses regular or stimulate abortion. Dr. Cheeseman's Pills, sold by mail order for $1 in the 1850s, were advertised in

70

Bloomington's *Weekly National Flag* to be:

> Mild in their operations, and certain to correct all irregu-
> larities, painful menstruation, removing all obstructions,
> whether from cold or otherwise, headache, pain in the side,
> palpitation of the heart, disturbed sleep, which always
> arise from interruption of nature. They can be successfully
> taken as a preventative. These pills should never be taken
> in pregnancy, as they would be sure to cause a
> miscarriage.[31]

Women were thought to be inherently weaker and more
subject to illness than men. Thus, many nostrums were marketed
to women as tonics with special powers to support unique female
processes and difficulties. The most famous and enduring of all of
these medicines was Lydia E. Pinkham's Vegetable Compound,
which first appeared on the market in the mid-1870s.[32] A
Massachusetts housewife, Lydia Estes Pinkham was 54 when the
Panic of 1873 brought economic hard times to her family. Mrs.
Pinkham had been accustomed to dosing her family and neighbors
with her own herbal remedies. One of these, adapted from a recipe
found in John King's *American Dispensatory*, became the
Vegetable Compound. It employed unicorn root to strengthen the
uterus and prevent miscarriage, and pleurisy root to cure prolapse.
These ingredients, together with life-root, black cohosh, fenugreek
seed and alcohol (approximately 18 percent of each bottle's con-
tents) went into the Compound.[33]

The Vegetable Compound promised to restore health and
vigor to tired, nervous women of all social classes. At the turn of
the century, one advertisement, pitched at working-class women,
said:

> "I am not well enough to work." How often these signifi-
> cant words are spoken in our great mills, shops, and facto-
> ries by the poor girl who has worked herself to the point
> where nature can endure no more and demands a rest! The
> poor sufferer, broken in health, must stand aside and make
> room for another. . . . Standing all day, week in and week
> out, or sitting in cramped positions, the poor girl has slowly
> contracted some deranged condition of her organic system,
> which calls a halt to her progress and demands restoration
> to health before she can be of use to herself or any one else.
> To this class of women and girls Mrs. Pinkham proffers
> both sympathy and aid. . . . We have on record thousands of
> such cases that have been absolutely and permanently

cured by Lydia E. Pinkham's Vegetable Compound. . . .[34]

Another, directed at upper-class women, described the "Tragedy" of society women "who brave death for social honors," working themselves into "nervous prostration" in the course of their social duties.[35]

Advertisements also catered to women's fear of the surgeon's knife. In one, used in about 1900, the headline proclaimed, "Operations Avoided":

> Hospitals in our great cities are sad places to visit. Three-fourths of the patients lying on those snow white beds are women and girls. Why should this be the case? Because they have neglected themselves. Every one of these patients had plenty of warning in these dragging sensations, pain at the left or right of side, nervous exhaustion, pain in the small of the back; all of which are indications of an unhealthy condition. Do not drag along at home or in your place of employment until you are obliged to go to the hospital and submit to an examination and possible operation. Build up the feminine system, remove the derangements which have signified themselves by danger signals, and remember that Lydia E. Pinkham's Vegetable Compound, made from native roots and herbs, has saved many women from the hospital.[36]

Advertisements from the 1920s and '30s reflect new concerns about female sexuality and psychology. Thus, the Compound promised to fuel women's sexual energy ("Men Love Peppy Girls"), support their wifely duties ("Are You Only a 3/4 Wife?"), and prevent nervous breakdown.[37] Pinkham's advertising slogan, "Only a woman understands a woman's ills," helped to develop a market which has endured into the late twentieth century, surviving governmental regulation, social changes and all evidence to the contrary regarding its claims of efficacy.

Wakefield's Medicine Factory

McLean County contributed to the national trade in patent medicines in the form of several locally manufactured nostrums, including Rue's Chloride of Gold and Wood Tar Compound, which promised to cure upper respiratory problems at the rate of sixty-four doses for fifty cents and was concocted and sold by Dr. G.H. Rue of Lexington.[38] The most well known local remedies, however, were manufactured by the Wakefield Medicine Factory, which was established in 1846. Indeed, Wakefield's Blackberry Balsam, a remedy for diarrhea, is still on sale in the 1990s.

Cyrenius Wakefield, born in 1815 in Watertown, New York, came to Illinois in 1837. Like many of the early migrants, he tried his hand at a number of trades. He taught school and farmed in both Blooming Grove and DeWitt County. However, his fortune was made with the arrival of his older brother, Zera, a physician who had developed a fever-cure during his ten years of medical practice in Arkansas. The brothers opened a store at Point Isabelle, DeWitt County, which profitably sold Zera's medicines. Indeed, so great was the demand that the brothers made plans to begin manufacturing the remedies. However, Zera Wakefield died in 1848, "leaving his brother sole owner of the business and his formulas."[39] Zera apparently also bequeathed his medical title to Cyrenius, who was known as Doctor Wakefield for the rest of his life.

In 1850, Cyrenius Wakefield moved to Bloomington and built a medicine factory and drug store, which he ran with his brother-in-law, Robert Thompson. He noted that he "sold from his little store to the amount of $2,000" in that year.[40] By 1857, the factory was so successful that Wakefield sold out his interest in the drug store and devoted his attention to manufacturing and advertising several patent medicines. He recruited agents, at first in the midwest, later nationally. In 1860, Wakefield's annual sales amounted to approximately $10,000. He bought a printing press and began publishing almanacs to advertise his products. In 1871, his son Oscar Wakefield and Oscar's brother-in-law C.S. Jones became partners in the firm. As of 1874:

> He [Cyrenius] gives employment to forty persons in his medicine business (one-half of whom are females) and his annual sales amount to $100,000. He converts twenty-five tons of paper into almanacs every year for free distribution, for the purpose of advertising his remedies. His largest sales are made where fevers are most dangerous and most common, particularly in new[ly settled] countries where he is glad to know that his remedies are the means of doing great good. . . . The Doctor has made himself quite independent by the judicious advertising of good and reliable remedies.[41]

During that period, these remedies included Wakefield's

Blackberry Balsam, Cathartic Liver Pills, Cherry Pectoral, Egyptian Salve, Golden Ointment, Resolvent, Rheumatic Resolvent, Worm Destroyer, Worm Lozenges and Wine Bitters.[42]

Like other nostrum manufacturers, Wakefield sold his products by testimonials, which were published in advertisements and literature distributed to salespeople. In an 1891 "Plain Statement," which was addressed "to the dealer," Wakefield's offered letters "from leading citizens of Bloomington and other places" indicating "why you should push our goods."[43] One letter, written by N.T. Cox of Leatherwood, Indiana, testified that:

> A five year old son of John Wildman of this place was sick with a cough for five months. Five different cough remedies were used, and also doctors' prescriptions, without relief. Then Wakefield's Cough Syrup was recommended, and they got one 25 cent bottle. They began giving it and saw a change, and when this was gone one 50 cent bottle was procured, which cured the child of consumption, which the doctors said he had.

Another, written by Mr. William Hawley Smith, "a distinguished citizen of Peoria, Illinois," said:

> GENTLEMEN — I write this to tell you how highly I prize your Blackberry Balsam as a remedy for diseases of the stomach and bowels. While traveling last summer I was taken with a very troublesome diarrhea, which followed me for some weeks, and finally compelled me to leave my business and return home. As soon as I reached Peoria, I placed myself under the care of a physician whom I have known for years, and who I have every reason to believe is one of the best practitioners in the state. He treated me for three weeks, without helping me a particle, and I began to fear that I was doomed to suffer for the rest of my life from Chronic Diarrhea. Finally I grew so weak that I was confined to the bed. While lying there, a friend induced me to try your Blackberry Balsam, since the doctor was not helping me. This I did, somewhat reluctantly I confess; but the very first dose I took of it "took hold", and before I had taken one bottle I was on my feet and able to resume my business. I think I took a part of a second bottle, but, anyhow, in a few days I was fully restored to health, and I have had no recurrence of the malady since that time. I believe

the medicine saved my life, and I take pleasure in thus rendering honor to whom honor is due.

Use of such testimonials was routine in the patent medicine trade. The format of these letters is typical, beginning with lingering illness, continuing with unsuccessful treatment by physicians and ending with triumphant use of the named remedy. Among other things, they indicate the nostrum-maker's eagerness for respectability and the overt tension between the official medical profession and the patent remedy industry.

In his prosperous later years, Cyrenius Wakefield became a pillar of the community. He was a member of the Bloomington Benevolent Society, the school board and the board of directors of People's Bank of Bloomington. He was active in the Republican party and friendly with Abraham Lincoln. He also enjoyed a prosperous lifestyle, which included construction of a "large stone residence" for the sum of approximately $30,000 in 1871, and extensive travel in the United States and Europe.[44] He died of pneumonia in 1885 which, according to legend, he contracted "while personally relieving cases of destitution."[45]

After his death, his family continued to operate the Wakefield Medicine Factory. In the twentieth century, its main product has been Blackberry Balsam, a diarrhea remedy containing blackberry root, white oak bark, columbo root, rhubarb root, culvers root, prickly ash bark, catechu gum, potassium carbonate, cranesbill, camphor and alcohol (12%). Blackberry Balsam is now manufactured and distributed by C. Wakefield & Company, located in Levittown, New York.

Conclusions

The late nineteenth century is often regarded as the heyday of the patent medicine trade. Technology, transportation and communication systems combined to support what had become a major capitalist enterprise, complete with robber barons and significant economic and political power. In comparison to Cyrenius Wakefield's relatively moderate success, other nostrum manufacturers operated on a truly grand scale. For instance, at the turn of the century, Charles Crittendon of New York stocked 12,000 proprietary remedies, "constantly acquiring and launching new brands of his own."[46] In 1881, the Proprietary Medicine Manufacturers and Dealers Association was established, becoming one of the first major lobbying organizations representing a commercial interest. The Association regulated trade practices among its members; it also resisted government initiatives to regulate the nostrum business.[47]

The market for over-the-counter remedies was stimulated by popular fascination with and expectations of science. People living in an era which had witnessed the triumphs of electricity, steam and distance communication had no trouble believing that new medicines could cure old diseases. Furthermore, scientific innovations were too new for people to have become very critical of them. For instance, the Anchor Electric Belt, which promised to cure rheumatism, liver and kidney disease, weak and lame back and other diseases, in addition to preventing colds and cold feet, was advertised at the same time that physicians were beginning to consider the diagnostic and therapeutic virtues of x-rays, first discovered in 1895.[48] Then as now, it was difficult to distinguish between technological miracles and quackery.

The patent medicine trade was also stimulated by the fact that, despite advances in biomedical science, few effective therapies existed for most of the ailments people suffered. While knowledge regarding killers like tuberculosis, heart disease and cancer had increased, no proven cures were available. Thus, sufferers and their families continued to buy patent remedies, hoping that these mixtures would succeed where the doctors had failed.

At the end of the nineteenth century, the patent medicine trade was enormously successful. However, its days of unregulated operation were numbered. Consumers were becoming increasingly urbanized and sophisticated. According to one authority, "Late nineteenth-century politics, transformed in orientation from party to issue affiliation, saw the number of voters increase massively and people beginning to use political processes to address their concerns."[49] One of these concerns was health.

Increasingly, consumers associated health standards with biomedical science, believing that the germs which caused diseases could be identified and eradicated with methods developed in laboratories. Patent remedy manufacturers took advantage of this trend, seeking to identify their products with medical authorities. For example, the name "Listerine" suggested both that the substance killed germs and that it was somehow associated with Dr. Joseph Lister who developed antiseptic surgical techniques. However, by the turn of the century, clever labeling was not sufficient to allay public concerns about the dangerous subtances used in many nostrums. Further, people began to care about whether nostrums could actually do what their manufacturers promised.

Public concern was encouraged by reformers such as the freelance journalist, Samuel Hopkins Adams, whose series, entitled "The Great American Fraud" appeared in *Colliers* magazine in 1905 and 1906. Adams wrote:

> Gullible Americans will spend this year some seventy-five million dollars in the purchase of patent medicines. In consideration of this sum it will swallow huge quantities of alcohol, an appalling amount of opiates and narcotics, a wide assortment of varied drugs ranging from powerful and dangerous heart depressants to insidious liver stimulants; and, far in excess of other ingredients, undiluted fraud. For fraud, exploited by the skilfulest of advertising bunco men, is the basis of the trade.[50]

Between 1904 and 1906, the *Ladies Home Journal* published articles by Mark Sullivan and Edward Bok, who educated consumers about the campaign against patent medicines. Like Upton Sinclair's expose on the meat-packing business, *The Jungle* (1906), such publications paved the way for the passage of legislation regulating the nostrum trade.

Even the Proprietary Medicine Association recognized that change was coming. In 1899, it agreed that some federal regulation should be imposed on the drug trade. In 1905, "In a secret meeting, the . . . Association urged the committee on legislation to work for a law that would exercise restraints on narcotics in nostrums, alcohol in patent medicines, and fraud in advertising."[51] Hence, both industry and public were prepared for the passage of the Pure Food and Drug Act in June, 1906. The Act required that specified ingredients, including alcohol, opiates, chloral hydrate, acetanilid, and several others, be stated on the product's label; that if the label said that certain ingredients (opiates, in particular) were not used, they must indeed not be present; and that false therapeutic claims for a remedy not be made.[52]

The Pure Food and Drug Act put an end neither to self-medication, nor to the patent medicine trade. As popular expectations regarding personal comfort increased, people took an increasing range of remedies and the drug business boomed. However, the 1906 Act did make over-the-counter preparations safer to use. Following a trend established by European governments, the federal government accepted as part of its responsibility guardianship of public safety — not only in foreign affairs, but within private homes. For the first time, unregulated use of narcotics became illegal. Physicians became the gatekeepers for these substances, as they would later be for antibiotics. The distinction between prescription and non-prescription drugs became a legal one. Accordingly, the Pure Food and Drug Act contributed both to the cause of public health and to the development of professional medicine.

5 Away From Home: Hospital Development

Introduction

The words "hospital" and "hospitality" share the same root. In traditional Europe, hospitals founded by religious and civil organizations offered shelter, sustenance and medical care to the needy. This hospitality was given without charge, as spiritually motivated charity which served the parallel purposes of rehabilitating the erring, housing the helpless and protecting the general population from contact with certain kinds of illnesses.[1] Both large urban hospitals, such as Paris's Hôtel Dieu and London's St. Bartholomew's, and smaller provincial institutions provided nursing, medical therapy and moral improvement to people unable to afford the more comfortable option of home care.

Hospital patients were housed in large wards, and often shared beds. Nursing was not a professional skill, but, rather, a personal service rendered by either nuns or servants, who also prepared and served food, cleaned wards and did the laundry. Ambulatory patients were usually expected to help with the work. Hospitals were run by matrons, under the general guidance of boards of governors or trustees. Admissions were often governed by wealthy patrons and usually dependent on the moral "worthiness" of the patient. The unworthy poor, such as syphilitics, alcoholics and pregnant prostitutes who were generally assumed to be suffering as the result of their own behavior, were often housed separately from more respectable patients.

While physicians, surgeons and apothecaries sometimes had voluntary or paid associations with hospitals, these associations were by no means usual. Indeed, medical therapy was a relatively insignificant part of hospital care, which emphasized diet, rest, prayer and regulated behavior. Before the late eighteenth century, hospitals were not used for medical education. Before the twentieth century, they were not typically used to house physicians' private patients. Indeed, before that time even patients paying for hospital accommodation were not separately charged for the doctor's attention. Thus, generally speaking, the rewards of medical practice were to be gained through attraction of a prosperous clientele — not through services rendered free to indigent hospital patients.[2]

Following the European model of rendering charitable care to the poor and others lacking access to home care, American hospitals were built beginning in colonial times. Military hospitals, isolation hospitals and at least one mental hospital, established at Williamsburg in 1773, served the needs of some special populations. More common were the almshouses erected in larger towns during the eighteenth century which provided shelter and custodial care to the destitute and chronically ill.[3]

In addition, rapidly growing American cities with their burgeoning immigrant populations recognized a need for hospitals providing medical care to the general public. In 1752, the Pennsylvania Hospital opened in Philadelphia. Like its European forebears, this institution existed primarily to serve the needs of the poor. However, heralding the unique direction which would be taken by American hospitals, it also admitted paying patients. [4]

Before the twentieth century, hospitals played a very small role in the provision of medical care. Virtually all births, illnesses, injuries and deaths were managed at home. Furthermore, no medical or surgical intervention had yet been devised which could not be administered at home as conveniently or safely as in a hospital. Most physicians' educations and careers progressed largely without association with hospitals. It is, therefore, not surprising that in 1873, the first American hospital survey identified only 178 hospitals in the nation.[5]

By the end of nineteenth century, this situation had begun to change. Throughout the United States, in maturing communities establishment of a hospital became a matter of local pride — a symbol of rectitude, prosperity and modernity. Associated with the popularization of the germ theory, adoption of antiseptic surgical techniques and the advent of technologies such as the x-ray, hospitals were visible monuments to scientific progress and enlightenment. In 1909, a census located 4,359 hospitals in the United States, exclusive of asylums for the mentally ill and sanitoria for the treatment of chronic diseases such as tuberculosis.[6]

Types of Hospitals

Three major types of hospitals developed in nineteenth-century America. The public hospital, operated on the basis of city or county funds, grew out of the almshouse tradition. Institutions such as Cook County in Chicago, Philadelphia General, Bellevue and Kings County in New York and San Francisco General hospitals, "were established as, and remained, institutions primarily for the very poor, and were associated with second-class social status and moral stigma."[7] While providing a necessary service, these hospitals had a bad reputation among the respectable public. The last resort of the homeless, indigent and vicious; chronically under-funded and over-crowded; hosts to apparently uncontrollable waves of infection; public hospitals were regarded as places no sensible person would go by choice.[8]

Proprietary hospitals were established by practitioners to house their own patients. As hospital care became more respectable and acceptable, and as surgery became safer and more lucrative, many small-town physicians built hospitals because such institutions were not otherwise locally available. Other doctors established small facilities, sometimes in their own homes, which catered to the fears and needs of middle-class patients who associated hospital care with dirt, discomfort and pauperization.[9] Some city physicians started their own hospitals out of frustration with the difficulty in obtaining access to often exclusive staff privileges in existing local hospitals. Approximately half of the American hospitals established by 1909 were privately owned.[10] Proprietary hospitals were profit-making ventures which may well have influenced the twentieth-century trend in favor of opening the staffs of charitable and religious hospitals to more physicians and allowing doctors to charge fees for services rendered to hospital patients.[11]

While the proportion of proprietary hospitals declined rapidly after 1920, due to financial pressures and physicians' perception that there were greater benefits in staff privileges than in ownership, these institutions helped establish a pattern in hospital development which distinguished the United States from other developed nations. Payment of fees entitled patients to home-like — even luxurious — accommodations. Hospitals serving private patients began, quite self-consciously, to model themselves upon hotels and to advertise accordingly.

The private charitable hospital, established either under nonsectarian community auspices or by religious organizations, became the dominant type in twentieth-century America. These institutions offered care without charge or at reduced rates to the poor, off-setting charity with fees from patients able to pay. Mustering support from churches, clubs, businesses and wealthy donors, charitable hospitals were viewed as exemplars of public service and altruism. Hospitals supported by religious groups — particularly Catholic and Jewish hospitals — also provided havens for immigrants who might be discriminated against or proselytized in hospitals run by the predominantly Protestant native-born population.[12]

As hospital care became acceptable among the middle and upper classes, the proportion of paying patients increased, in turn supporting the general principle of payment for hospital services. No contradiction was observed between the notion of the hospital as a charitable institution and that of payment for hospital care. Indeed, at the Columbian Exposition in 1893, Arthur Ryerson, president of Chicago's St. Luke's Hospital, advocated the pay system as the "true scientific plan" for hospital charity.[13]

Paying patients received better accommodations than charity patients. Thus, it was not uncommon for hospital buildings to reflect the developing two-tiered system of care, with private patients inhabiting private rooms with attached baths and sometimes sitting- rooms, while charity patients were cared for in large common wards. Since early twentieth-century hospitals stays were often very long, the environment of care was important in regards to both the patient's comfort and the family's decision to opt for hospital rather than home care.

Hospital Management

Early nineteenth-century American hospitals were run by matrons, under the supervision of boards of trustees. Not until the end of the century would physicians assume the responsibility and power of administrative decision-making. The day-to-day work of hospitals was done by untrained nurses, servants and ambulatory patients. Ward staff members and patients tended to share the same lowly social and economic status. The public hospitals of the eastern cities were crowded, dirty and unruly. Profanity, theft and drunkenness abounded. Specifically opposed to admission of the acutely or terminally ill, these institutions were refuges for patients suffering from chronic diseases, who often remained for years. Lacking external means of support, patients often migrated between hospital and almshouse. Hospitals were composed of large common wards. Without specially designated spaces for examinations, surgical operations, childbirth or death, there was little privacy or protection from the sights, sounds and odors associated with suffering and care.

The 1844 journal kept by John Duffe, a ward nurse and possible ex-patient in New York Hospital's Marine House, offers a glimpse of contemporary working conditions:

He was an experienced dresser of wounds and infections, and administered countless baths and enemas. At the same time, and with occasional help from the healthier patients, he scrubbed the floors, washed the sheets, fetched dinner for the men on the ward. And until the hospital arranged to have the city's new water supply introduced in pipes throughout the building, much of his work consisted of "carrying and luging [sic] of Slops and all kinds of filth and dirt." On those rare days when he received "liberty," Duffe had to find a patient healthy and reliable enough to substitute for him. "So ends this days work," he noted at the close of one long day, "for work we may call it without end."[14]

Although he could not have known it, Duffe's labors were performed at the end of a long era. Hospitals were about to undergo an enormous change.

This change was generated, in part, by publicity regarding the results of Florence Nightingale's reorganization of British military hospitals during the Crimean War (1854-6). Nightingale used statistics to show that the introduction of order, cleanliness and nourishing diets reduced mortality rates and lengths of hospital stays, returning more soldiers to their regiments more quickly. Her methods were copied by Americans including Dorothea Dix, Clara Barton and "Mother" Mary Ann Bickerdyke during the Civil War, inaugurating a period of hospital reform. New hospitals were built with wards designed for ventilation and cleanliness. These hospitals increasingly housed nurse-training schools where respectable young women found that virtue and nursing were not incompatible.

Between the late nineteenth century and the 1940s, student nurses did most of the day-to-day work of American hospitals not run by religious orders.[15] Nurse training took the form of practical apprenticeship enhanced by minimal academic instruction. Student nurses took over the work formerly done by untrained nurses and servants. They scrubbed floors, made beds, did laundry, served meals, emptied slops and made the bandages, plasters and cotton swabs not yet available in disposable form. They also performed most hands-on patient care. Graduate nurses tended to opt for better-paid private duty nursing. Only after World War II, when the escalation of medical technology required increasing nursing expertise, and the development of intensive care facilities put an end to the need for private duty nurses, did academic nurse training replace apprenticeship and professional registered nurses replace students in hospital work.[16]

The changing relationship between physicians and hospitals relates to the increased utilization of urban hospitals for clinical teaching, the increasing importance of access to laboratory facilities and medical equipment, and the development of medical specialties. With escalating use of hospital facilities in the late nineteenth century, particularly for surgical operations, physicians became increasingly interested in obtaining staff privileges. Also, as members of community elites, doctors became increasingly involved in the organization of new hospitals. New public confidence in the potential of official medical treatment lent physicians new authority. Hospital medical staffs became increasingly powerful in setting hospital policies and planning hospital development.

As middle class patients became willing to receive care in hospitals, physicians discovered that attending their patients in hospitals was far more convenient and efficient than visiting them in their homes. Under pressure from medical staffs, hospitals purchased expensive equipment such as x-ray machines, operating room tables and laboratory paraphernalia. They also reorganized internal space to accommodate the demands of specialists for surgical and obstetrical facilities, and separate areas for children and people suffering from infectious diseases. With the development of a rapidly expanding array of medical specialty board examinations after 1920, hospitals became the professional homes of specialists who increasingly dominated medical staffs and hospital decision-making. By 1940, almost one quarter of American physicians were full-time specialists, with many more adding a part-time specialty to general practice.[17] In 1966, 69 percent of practicing physicians were specialists; in 1969, nearly one third of the profession was composed of surgical specialists.[18]

The late nineteenth century witnessed the birth of a new profession — hospital administration. In 1899, administrators founded an Association of Hospital Superintendents, which in 1908 changed its name to the American Hospital Association. As hospital functions grew more specialized and complicated, and as hospital finances became more challenging, a new level of expertise was required to operate these institutions. The development of professional hospital administration paralleled the growth of physicians' authority over hospital management. However, in the mid-twentieth century, medical domination of hospitals weakened and the authority of administrators grew, largely as a result of the need for integration of the growing array of hospital functions and the emphasis on the hospital as a business operation.[19]

Regional Developments

The foundation of hospitals in the Midwest followed migration and population growth. Only a small village in 1830, by the 1870s Chicago supported a range of hospitals including Mercy (1850), Cook County (1865), Chicago Hospital for Women and Children (1865), the Illinois Charitable Eye and Ear Hospital (1866), and the Woman's Hospital of the State of Illinois (1871). Other Illinois communities built hospitals as their size and prosperity made this possible.

Caring for the Ailing Poor

In Illinois at the turn of the twentieth century, relatively few counties made formal provision for medical care of the indigent, depending instead upon arrangements with local charitable hospitals for the care of the acutely ill poor. With the exception of Cook County Hospital, with its resident medical staff offering a full range of services, most counties offered only the limited resources of poor houses or county farms. According to one expert, these facilities "were characterized by filth, flies, no shades or screens, no medical attendants or nurses, with the insane kept in iron-barred cages — conditions that would exist in some rural areas throughout the United States well into the 1920s, and probably well beyond."[20]

McLean County was typical of Illinois counties in not establishing a public hospital. While the County began to make public provision for the care of the indigent in the 1850s, the ailing poor were not distinguished from their able-bodied brethren. After hospital development began in 1880, both inmates of the Poor Farm, established in 1860, and other impoverished County inhabitants, received hospital care partially paid for out of County funds. Despite some discussion in the 1880s of building an insane asylum on Poor Farm property, no specific institutional provision was made for publicly funded care of either the mentally or physically ill.[21]

In 1914 the McLean County Poor Farm was criticized by an inspector from the Illinois Charities Commissions for housing its inmates in unsanitary, vermin-ridden and foul-smelling buildings, and for leaving the care of the frail elderly and chronically ill entirely to other residents.[22] The inspector advocated the establishment of a hospital ward at the Poor Farm, claiming that this would be more cost effective than the prevailing practice of contracting with local hospitals for the care of acutely ill inmates. However, this argument was countered by the county physician, Dr. DaCosta, who maintained that, since the hospitals picked up about half of the daily cost of caring for County patients, construction of a separate facility at the Poor Farm would be unrealistic, representing an unnecessary expense to taxpayers. While Poor Farm buildings were old, a 1916 visit by County Board members found them clean and adequate for the use of residents.

In 1925, the Poor Farm's population reached its peak of 123 inmates. For a time during the mid-twentieth century, it did operate a sixteen-bed hospital ward. However, the number of residents declined steadily, and the ward closed when World War II began, creating local shortages in medical practitioners. Always run at a loss, annual deficits grew and the property became increasingly dilapidated:

> By the end of World War II . . . its population had dwindled to thirty, and the buildings were deteriorating badly. The Poor Farm had become a shelter for derelicts, hoboes and the insane. The sleeping rooms contained the bare necessities and looked much like a typical jail cell. The living quarters were dark, dreary and smelly places that were both unsafe and poorly equipped. [23]

In the early 1950s, the Farm's population had shrunk to between ten and fifteen inmates at any one time. It closed in 1954, to be replaced by the McLean County Nursing Home, for twenty years operating in the renovated Poor Farm residence building, and after 1974 occupying a purpose-built structure in north Normal.[24]

Hospitals in McLean County

St. Joseph's Hospital

While McLean County never established a public hospital, it was otherwise typical in nurturing both charitable and proprietary hospitals. St. Joseph's Hospital was founded in 1880 in Bloomington by five Sisters belonging to the Third Order of St. Francis in Peoria. The Sisters asked Dr. Charles Ross Parke, an established Bloomington surgeon, to select a "medical staff that would work in perfect harmony."[25] That this Catholic charitable hospital should be historically first was appropriate, since "Illinois reported the largest cluster of Roman Catholic hospitals of any state" at the turn of the century — 43 out of a total of 118 hospitals.[26] Members of a German nursing order driven from their own country by Otto von Bismarck's anti-Catholic policies, the nuns who ran St. Joseph's Hospital retained close contact with members of their order, both in other parts of the United States and in Germany. Indeed, German women continued to be recruited for service in the order's American hospitals in the mid-twentieth century.[27]

Quickly outgrowing its initial accommodation in what had been the east-side home of Mr. Samuel W. Waddle, St. Joseph's Hospital expanded in 1883 and 1888. After purchase of three city blocks, an east wing was added in 1908. An addition on the west side was made in 1920, followed by a building to house the School of Nursing, accredited in 1921. Indeed, no fewer than eight additions were made to the original hospital building before it was replaced with a new building in 1966.

Kelso Sanitarium and Fuller Clinic

The foundation of St. Joseph's Hospital was followed in 1894 with the establishment of the proprietary Bloomington Home Sanitarium by Doctors George and Annie Kelso.[28] As homeopaths, the Kelsos received a rather chilly reception from the County's allopathic medical establishment.[29] Thus, possession of their own hospital made possible the full exercise of their specialties, George's in surgery and Annie's in obstetrics. The hospital, later renamed the Kelso Sanitarium, was so successful that by 1916 it had 85 rooms and 60 patient beds. Marketed to the prosperous, including "the nerve-racked business man" and "the woman grown weary of social demands," the Sanitarium served as a local alternative to charitable hospitals, where both desperate illness and poverty might be encountered.[30] Prospective patients were promised "the comforts and quietness of a club or home" where "one week . . . of enjoyable health building is worth many weeks of exciting amusement at seashore or resort."[31] Like other local hospitals, the Sanitarium operated a nurse training school. The Kelsos sold the Sanitarium building to the Mennonite Sanitarium Association in 1920, thereafter operating a smaller hospital and clinic next to their home.

Dr. Annie Kelso died in 1927. Dr. George Kelso kept the hospital and clinic open for a short time thereafter, but decided to retire in about 1930. He sold his home and the nine-bed hospital building on the corner of Main and Chestnut streets to Dr. Fuller, an osteopath, who operated what was then called the Fuller Clinic until World War II made it difficult to find nurses. The Clinic "was an osteopathic clinic and a full hospital with operating facilities and everything." [32] According to Dr. Fuller's daughter,

> He had a medical doctor in with him and they did full oper-
> ations — I don't mean they did research things or anything
> like that. Appendectomies and all kinds of abdominal
> things and the regular . . . general surgery. They did that
> until the place caught on fire [mid-1930s]. He never did re-
> institute the surgical part of it. He still had it for pneumo-
> nia cases and broken bones and all sorts of things of that
> sort, but not surgery.

Patients at the Fuller Clinic paid approximately nine dollars per day for accommodation, which included private rooms and meals prepared by an excellent German cook.[33] Two nurses cared for them. While the Clinic was never regarded as a rest home, several elderly patients stayed there for long periods of time. Indeed, many patients apparently required minimal care because Dr. Fuller encouraged them to go home on weekends — a policy which had the unforeseen benefit of leaving the hospital virtually empty when it caught on fire one Sunday evening in July. After the hospital closed in the 1940s, it was converted to an apartment building.

Brokaw Hospital

In 1896, with financial support from five local doctors and several Mennonite churches, the Deaconess Hospital opened. This charitable hospital, established as the Protestant alternative to the existing Catholic facility, was more successful in attracting patients than in generating continuing support from Mennonite organizations. In its first year, the twenty-bed facility was staffed by Mennonite deaconesses. However, in 1897, their contract with the hospital was discontinued for the following religious reasons:

> In hospital work the power and wisdom of man is shown
> forth rather than that of Christ and hence He does not get

the glory. And since His glory is the aim of our work, we can not cooperate in a work where this aim cannot be reached.[34]

Between 1897 and 1902, nursing was performed by members of a Methodist Deaconess Society, who also apparently began to teach student nurses.[35]

Demand for hospital beds quickly outgrew the available accommodations; plans for a new building began in 1898. However, despite strenuous fundraising activities, sufficient funds were lacking. Then, in 1901 a local businessman, Abram Brokaw, contributed $10,000 to the hospital, which was renamed in his honor. In 1903, Brokaw sold his plow factory and used the proceeds to establish an endowment fund for the hospital. The substantial bequest of $100,000 and two 160-acre farms after Brokaw's death in 1905 helped to ensure the hospital's continuing financial stability. A second hospital building was opened in 1904, making possible the accommodation of a nurse training school. In 1909 a nurses home was built, and in 1913 a third hospital building opened. The hospital expanded with construction of a new nurses home, the May Mecherle Hall, in 1941, and additions in 1953, 1956 and 1967.

Mennonite Hospital

Toward the end of World War I, interest among local Mennonite leaders in establishing a hospital revived. According to Rev. Emanual Troyer, a champion of this project, there were some early doubts:

> Rev. Kinsinger [of Danvers] was one who was luke warm toward the project. He felt the group assembled, being mostly farmers, didn't know a thing about running a hospital. I said to him that when the war was on, we went to the government to see if the Mennonite boys could do some work in the military without carrying guns. This concession was made and now the war is over and the government is asking us, "What do you do now when the war is over? Are you active only in time of war, or is your testimony for help and caring even when there is no emergency?" Seeing the wisdom of this, Rev. Kinsinger became quite active in supporting the hospital.[36]

The Mennonite Sanitarium Association was formed in 1919 with the purpose of establishing a hospital, sanitarium and nurse training school in Bloomington. In 1920, the Association purchased the Kelso Sanitarium and Training School, together with most of its equipment, for $75,000. The eleven student nurses already enrolled in the Kelso Training School stayed on, becoming the first graduates of the Mennonite Sanitarium Training School.

Like other local hospitals, Mennonite experienced space shortages, and initiated an expansion project every decade from 1931 to 1981. With the original Kelso Sanitarium building at its center, additions were built in 1932, 1941, 1956, 1969, 1970 and 1981. In 1946, student nurses obtained their own housing and educational facilities when the Troyer Memorial Nurses Home was completed.

Other Hospitals in the County

Beginning in the 1880s, Bloomington served as McLean County's medical center. While small communities in rural areas invariably enjoyed the services of physicians, dentists, druggists and midwives, their residents generally traveled to Bloomington if hospital care was needed. Indeed, a 1920 promotional pamphlet for Brokaw Hospital recognized the regional nature of the hospital's market:

> Brokaw Hospital should not be considered strictly a
> Bloomington and Normal institution. It receives patients
> from any locality, and its records show an increasing
> patronage each year by people who live in the country and
> small Illinois towns who wish to avail themselves of this
> institution for medical or surgical treatment. The central
> location of Bloomington, its excellent railroad and interur-
> ban service makes Brokaw Hospital especially desirable by
> patients, their families and their family physician who may
> wish to make frequent visits to the institution. Patients
> living outside of Bloomington and Normal will have the
> same care and consideration that any local person would
> have and we invite them to avail themselves of the hospital
> service.

However, rural residents were slower than their urban counterparts to use hospitals on a routine basis. One oral history respondent, born in 1906, said of his neighbors in his hometown of

90

Lexington, "I never knew of anybody going to the hospital. . . . When people died, they died in their homes."[37] Until the mid-twentieth century, rural residents gave birth and received most of their medical treatment, including surgery, in their homes. When they did require hospitalization, this involved a long journey and often a long stay at some distance from family and friends.

This situation was inconvenient for both patients and physicians. Thus, in 1921 Dr. L.M. Johnson built a small hospital in Arrowsmith to serve his own patients. He operated the hospital until his death in 1948. Thereafter, the building was used as an apartment, a nursing home, and a private home.[38] Similarly, the only hospital in Woodford County, Eureka Hospital, was founded in 1901, and used by several local doctors in succession. Purchased in 1978 by the Mennonite Hospital Association, Eureka Community Hospital together with BroMenn Regional Medical Center and BroMenn/Lifecare Center, is now part of BroMenn Healthcare.[39]

Instead of opening a general hospital, Dr. F.J. Parkhurst of Danvers specialized in the treatment of problem drinkers. An active temperance advocate, he founded the Willow Bark Institute in 1892.[40] The Willow Bark Cure was based on frequent administration of a bitter vegetable-based liquid, the main ingredient of which was salicin, a colorless water-soluble glycoside obtained from the bark of the willow tree. Patients were encouraged to associate this remedy with strong drink, thus losing their taste for alcohol. In 1902, Dr. Parkhurst built the Concord Hotel to house his patients. The Hotel burned in 1907, and the Willow Bark Institute in 1908. Thereafter, the doctor accommodated patients in his own home until 1920. In 1935, the Willow Bark Cure was revived by Mr. and Mrs. Ernest Mammen, who treated patients in the Parkhurst home until they retired in 1950.[41]

With the exception of the Willow Bark Institute, the institutions discussed above represent the major trends in American hospital development. All full-service medical facilities, they grew as the result of increasing patient acceptance of hospital treatment; increasing dependence upon hospital environments and technology for many kinds of treatment; and the increasing role of the hospital as the site for treatment rendered by the growing number of medical specialists.

Hospital Management and Finances

Until the second half of the twentieth century, the three

major charitable hospitals in McLean County were run by people without formal hospital administration qualifications. Hospital management structures reflected their historical roots and organizational affiliations. St. Joseph's Hospital, for instance, was administered by a Mother Superior, who managed communication with her order's headquarters in Peoria, dealt with the hospital's medical staff, and supervised the work of nursing Sisters, student nurses (after 1921) and other hospital employees. Although by the mid-twentieth century the hospital employed professionally qualified lay administrators, ultimate direction still rests with the nine members of the Third Order of St. Francis Healthcare's governing board, seven of whom are nuns.[42]

Until the late 1950s, Mennonite Hospital was run by married couples referred to as the Superintendent and Matron. The hospital's second Superintendent, Noble Hoover, had been a farmer and electrician before he was hired by Mennonite in 1927 because of his "business experience". In addition to dealing with the desperate financial challenges facing the hospital during the Depression, "He took a working interest in all operations of the hospital work, soon learning to take x-rays so he could relieve the only x-ray technician during the nights, every other Sunday, and holidays."[43] In 1934, he "devised a plan for making ice packs by a formula of alcohol, ether and water. He put this mixture in hot water bags where it became cold and slushy, making an ice bag that fitted to the contour of the patient's body."[44] Esther Hoover became the business office manager, receptionist and supervisor of the hospital's housekeeping, laundry and kitchen staff. Having weathered the enormous changes caused by debt, expansion, medical specialization and the introduction of hospital insurance, the Hoovers retired in 1956. Thereafter, Mennonite's administrators have all had professional qualifications.[45]

Before 1924, Brokaw Hospital and its School for Nurses shared a Superintendent, who was responsible to the Board of Directors for cost-effective management of the day-to-day work of the hospital. Early Superintendents were graduate nurses with some experience in hospital and nursing administration. In a revealing 1939 comment, Maude Essig said of Miss Lula Justis, Superintendent between 1907 and 1924:

> She was a most economical manager and was a valuable assistant to the Board of directors in helping to pay off the bonded indebtedness on the new building. This she did perhaps at the expense, sometimes, of patients' comfort,

since it is a generally recognized fact that one cannot take in from patients more than enough to meet the actual running expenses of the hospital and in most hospitals the latter is impossible.[46]

In 1924, Miss Essig became the first separate director of Brokaw's School of Nursing.

Hospital finances were always a challenge, despite the growing demand for hospital treatment. Unlike the proprietary hospitals, which were intended to be profit-making concerns, during the first half of the twentieth century charitable institutions kept charges low for paying patients and, regardless of financial pressures, continued to treat a significant number of patients without charge. In 1930, for example, Brokaw hospital admitted 2,758 patients, accounting for a total of 22,378 patient days of treatment. Of this total, 67 patient days were provided free, and 82 percent of patients were treated for sums under the $4.99 reckoned to be the daily per capita cost of hospital care.[47] Thus, despite the fact that payments received from patients provided the lion's share of hospitals' incomes, with ever increasing operating expenses, debts to pay, and expansion campaigns, hospitals struggled to remain solvent.

All three hospitals depended heavily upon local fundraising campaigns. Early St. Joseph's records indicate that, in addition to regular collections and occasional large contributions (in January 1882, for example, a Mr. Flanagan gave $1,000 which was laid aside for the planned new building), the Sisters went from door to door requesting money from homes and workplaces; received donations of food and clothing; and held raffles.[48] Initiating a pattern followed by other local hospitals, St. Joseph's named rooms in its 1909 addition for major individual and organizational donors.

Before Abram Brokaw became its patron, Deaconess Hospital had considerable trouble raising money to cover operating expenses and plans for expansion. The Building Committee resorted to direct appeals for donations and benefit entertainments. "The outstanding performances given to raise money in 1898 were a 'Barbeque' and 'District Skule,' the two netting about $1,800."[49] Even after the institution became Brokaw Hospital, community support was very important. Charity Balls were held, and members of organizations including local churches, the Ladies' Aid Society (later supplanted by the Women's Service League), and the Home Bureau raised money, made in-kind donations, and volunteered in the hospital. In 1920, Brokaw's promotional booklet made very clear its dependence upon community support:

> Brokaw Hospital depends largely on the revenue derived
> from its patients, the present endowment fund providing
> but a small part of the necessary amount for it to operate.
> The moderate rates which are charged the patients and the
> great amount of free work done make the income of this
> institution wholly inadequate to accumulate any consider-
> able sinking fund for future expansion. Gifts or bequests
> from those who appreciate the great work that this institu-
> tion is doing will be highly appreciated and expended for
> new buildings, equipping rooms or adding to the general
> fund as the donor may desire.

Mennonite Hospital initially depended upon investments
made by individual members of the Hospital Association and contributions, both financial and in-kind, from Mennonite churches.
For example, on Thanksgiving Day, 1921, the following items were
received from churches:

> 12 gallons of lard, 7 bushels of potatoes, 2 bushels of apples,
> 1 1/4 bushels of carrots, 2 bushels of onions, 4 dozen eggs,
> 30 heads of cabbage, 5 chickens, 1 turkey, 70 glasses of jelly,
> 1 box of homemade soap, 3 dozen bunches of celery, 440
> quarts of fruit, and 1 quarter of beef.[50]

Despite loyal support from both churches and individuals, however, Mennonite apparently had more economic problems than the
other hospitals. In early years, there were "occupancy problems"
attributed to rivalry with the older hospitals and the tendency of
general practitioners to refer patients to specialists with staff privileges at these other hospitals.[51] While this situation improved
somewhat in the early 1930s after Dr. Edwin P. Sloan (1878-1935)
moved most of his goiter surgery from St. Joseph's to Mennonite,
patients' own financial problems discouraged hospital use during
the Depression.[52] Nonetheless, by 1932 the hospital, which had
just erected a new addition, was so deeply in debt that all employees went on half pay, and creditors formed a creditors' committee
to try to secure their interests. In 1935,

> One firm went so far as to have its attorney and another
> representative, together with the sheriff, back a truck up to
> the back door of the hospital. They were going to carry out

furniture until they obtained enough to satisfy their claim. Hoover [the Superintendent] went out to them and said, "Now, you can do this. I can't prevent you. But before you do it, I think you ought to know that there are a dozen or more other companies who have just the same claim as you have, and back of them is a group of bondholders who hold a mortgage on all this hospital real estate and all the furnishings of this institution. Now, you could take this out, but you might have to prove in court that you had a prior right." Apparently they weren't sure they could prove their claim, so they left without any furniture.[53]

Finally, in 1936, the hospital was refinanced, a settlement was made with its creditors, and Mennonite began to look forward to a period of prosperity and expansion.

In the mid-twentieth century, Bloomington's hospitals engaged in increasingly ambitious fundraising. In 1949, St. Joseph's and Mennonite conducted a joint campaign which raised $350,000. In 1955, Mennonite received a $63,700 grant from the Ford Foundation. In the 1960s, Mennonite, Brokaw and St. Joseph's joined the large number of community hospitals in Illinois which received building grants under the Hill-Burton Act — legislation passed in 1946 which recognized the growing importance of hospital care by authorizing a major program of federal grants to states to aid construction of hospitals.[54]

All local hospitals benefited from the boom in hospitalization which began in the late 1930s. By this time, hospitals had metamorphosed, from places poor people went to die, to treatment factories where the latest scientific techniques were employed to banish ill-health. Care of acute or serious illness moved from homes to institutions and from lay to professional supervision. "Occupancy rates for general hospitals rose from 64 percent in 1935 to 70 percent in 1940 — rates much higher than in the late 1920s — while the average length of stay decreased."[55] Hospitalization became a recognized necessity. With burgeoning medical technology and proliferation of hospital-based specialists, it also became increasingly expensive.

In 1935, charitable hospitals in the United States received 71 percent of their income from patients.[56] However, particularly during those economically difficult times, it was a continual struggle for providers to collect from patients and their families. Prepayment plans became an increasingly attractive alternative for both hospitals and the communities they served. Group hospital-ization insurance plans, soon identified with Blue Cross, guaran-teed hospital care to subscribers and payment to the hospitals they used. As insurance coverage became more common, hospital utilization increased.

Also stimulating demand for hospital beds was the avail-ability of antibiotics after World War II. This development made surgery safer than it had ever been before, thus encouraging increasingly frequent and ambitious procedures. It also facilitated the speedy treatment and cure of diseases which previously had required extensive periods of bed rest and nursing care. Having spent the first half of the twentieth century extracting themselves from home-based consultations, physicians divided their practices between their offices and the hospitals (usually more than one) with which they were affiliated. As the site for both surgery and the treatment of acute infection, the hospital's popularity and prestige sky-rocketed.

Hospital Services

McLean County's early hospitals offered very different ser-vices from those they currently provide. Without specific drug therapies, illnesses lasted a very long time. Hospitals mainly offered skilled nursing care and surgical facilities. Indeed, before the 1920s, hospitals were generally thought to be useful primarily for surgical operations. Even in the early twentieth century, many patients and doctors continued to opt for home surgery. Thus, in its 1916 advertising pamphlet, the Kelso Sanitarium both praised the quality of its surgical facilities and argued in favor of hospital rather than home treatment:

> With the completed addition of our new surgical pavilion,
> we now have one of the most splendidly equipped surgical
> departments in the State. . . . Our operating rooms are sup-
> plied with every surgical appliance for all lines of surgical
> work. The sterilizing rooms adjoining are fitted with the
> latest devices for sterilizing dressings, instruments, uten-
> sils and clothing. . . . Hundreds of critical operations are
> performed in this department every year with results
> which would not be possible without the advantages of the
> special preparation and "after" care to which the particular
> personal attention of the surgeon is given.

All local hospitals marketed themselves on the basis of their surgical facilities. In 1920, Brokaw hospital boasted five operating rooms; nine of its 24 medical staff members were surgeons.[57] In 1931, Mennonite Hospital admitted 891 patients and performed over 600 surgical operations.[58]

Presence on a hospital staff of a surgeon with a good reputation and an unusual specialty could be enormously beneficial to the hospital. Such a surgeon attracted referrals and filled hospital beds. Thus, Mennonite Hospital profited from "the continued efforts of E.P. Sloan. Many goiter patients came to Mennonite Sanitarium from all over Illinois and Kentucky to receive his care. Dr. Sloan often had as many as five goiter surgeries in one day at the hospital." When Dr. Sloan was "in Europe continuing his goiter work," hospital occupancy dropped. Mennonite also nurtured the work in orthopedic surgery of Dr. Herman W. Wellmerling (1887-1979) and in eye surgery of Dr. Watson Gailey (1882-1959), profiting from both their reputations and their patients.[59]

Indeed, so strongly associated with surgery was hospital care that hospitals made a deliberate attempt to market their other services. Brokaw Hospital's 1920 promotional pamphlet argued that, in addition to operating rooms, its facilities provided a better environment for care of internal illnesses than patients' homes:

> Many people have the mistaken idea that a hospital is solely for surgical cases. More and more each year the hospital is receiving cases where the best medical attention, scientific nursing, proper diet, perfect rest and everything possible is done to restore the patient to normal health. Caring for the sick in the average home is a burden to the family, and with the most loving care of the home folks a patient cannot have the scientific treatment and sanitary surroundings, and plainly speaking does not have the chance for a quick and complete recovery that he would have in a modern equipped hospital.

In addition to the therapies for acute illnesses provided by hospitals, sanitariums offered aids to health incorporating a variety of treatments, including dietary management, massage, electricity and baths. In 1916, the Kelso Sanitarium offered "Sitz, Steam, Needle and Shower baths, Electric Light, electric water and electric robe baths, salt glows, oil rubs, hot packs, fomentations, [and] Scotch douches" to support the health and beauty of clients who checked in for rest, recreation and rejuvenation. Massage facilities included exercise machines (called "mechanical massage") designated for the use of chronic invalids. Electricity was administered to patients by means of "the newest and most approved apparatus. . . in order that each patient might have that particular current which would be of most benefit." Baths, massages and electrical treatments continued to be provided at Mennonite Hospital during the 1920s and early 1930s, but were discontinued in 1933 when the Bath Department had become unprofitable.[60]

In early years, sanitariums and hospitals also provided long-term care. Unlike the Poor Farm, which housed seniors without financial or family resources, local hospitals became the home of choice for some middle-class people who found them more comfortable than private accommodation. Thus, in August 1884, Mrs. Kath Weismuller paid St. Joseph's Hospital $410 for a "home for life." When she died in October 1897, the hospital paid $35 for her burial. During the same period other elderly people paid smaller weekly or monthly sums for their "board" in the hospital.[61]

The Fuller Clinic housed at least one long-term resident during the 1930s. Grandma Poulton, in her late eighties, had been brought to the hospital with pneumonia:

> She loved it there. Her family loved her very much, but I
> imagine she was a great deal of care. And she was very
> happy there. The family just wondered if she couldn't stay,
> because she ate better there, the nurses got her up and
> made her walk and do things out in the yard. And we did
> have Grandma Poulton for about a year and a half until she
> passed away.[62]

Mrs. Poulton's family paid approximately $9 per week to keep her at the Fuller Clinic.

In 1936, Mr. John L. Lampe made arrangements with the Board of Directors for a permanent home and care in Brokaw hospital, after which he occupied "Room 109 in exchange for some real estate and securities." During his stay, Lampe improved the hospital's amenities, paying for installation of new wall sockets and light fixtures in all of the old building's rooms, improving the patients' call system, having a new bath tub installed in the Men's room and purchasing a gasoline powered lawn mower.[63]

Mennonite Hospital had provided long-term care in the old

Kelso Sanitarium building until 1931, when that building was torn down. In 1970, a new formal program was instituted when 38 patient beds were designated for nursing the aged. So popular was this unit that its capacity was doubled in 1971. In 1974, an adult day care program was added to Mennonite's long-term care services.[64]

Early hospitals recognized that many poor people in the community could neither afford medical care nor spend time in hospitals. Thus, they sent nurses into the community to treat patients in their own homes. Beginning in 1905, Brokaw Hospital employed a visiting nurse "whose duties were to visit the homes of the sick and render service where their circumstances did not permit their paying for it." In 1906, the nurse visited 161 patients, making a total of 2,415 calls. She delivered 14 babies and assisted at three surgical operations. Only 12 patients were sent to the hospital.[65] Brokaw stopped administering the service in 1920, when the City of Bloomington assumed this role.[66]

Like medicine generally, hospitals changed with the introduction of new technologies, medical specialties and popular expectations regarding health, illness and medical care. Early hospitals were general hospitals, without areas specially designated for the care of specific categories of patients. One major early innovation was the establishment of obstetrical facilities and wards. Before 1920, most McLean County babies were born at home. However, with increased concern about germs in the early years of the twentieth century, and increased confidence in professional medical expertise, the trend, led by middle-class mothers, was in favor of hospital deliveries. The Kelso Sanitarium recognized this market, advertising in 1916:

> In order to meet this trying and critical period with more
> success, we have fitted rooms especially for this purpose.
> They are large, sunny and furnished in pleasing taste.
> There is an aseptic delivery room in connection which is
> completely equipped. . . . The fact that every detail can be
> carried out under the supervision of the physician makes it
> in every way more desirable and much more satisfactory to
> the patient [than home confinement]. We believe that our
> success in the handling of this class of patients is due to the
> fact that our physicians deeply appreciate this delicate con-
> dition and every attention is given and alert vigilance
> observed in order that the mothers may have a minimum of
> stress and a better chance for an excellent recovery. This

plan relieves the mother of all domestic and social cares during her seclusion and convalescence, and results in a more satisfactory return to health and a more correct beginning for the child.

The three local charitable hospitals followed Kelso's lead, by 1920 considering obstetrical services an integral part of their functions. An early medical specialty, with board certification established in 1930, obstetrics involved increasing use of anesthetics, technical equipment and surgery, all more conveniently available in hospitals. By 1939, half of all American mothers and 75% of urban mothers were delivering in hospitals.[67] Demand for hospital-based obstetrical services mushroomed during the Baby Boom following World War II, leading to expansion in all local obstetrical departments. However, by the 1960s the number of births began to decline. A cooperative study of local capacity and needs sponsored by Brokaw, St. Joseph's and Mennonite hospitals led to the closure of Mennonite's obstetrical unit in 1968.[68] Since that time, the hospitals have specialized, with Brokaw becoming the first hospital in the area to have birthing rooms, while in 1983 St. Joseph's received a special designation from the State of Illinois to treat unhealthy newborns of intermediate risk.

In addition to obstetrical services, local hospitals also added pediatric units in the mid-twentieth century. Before that time, ailing children had been cared for in their homes. However, with increasingly routine surgery, such as tonsillectomy, performed on children, hospitals responded to the demand for facilities.

With their specialized equipment, hospitals also became centers for treatment of infantile paralysis, or polio, the first major epidemic of which struck the eastern United States in 1916, and became a significant threat to health in McLean County in the 1920s. Prior to 1946, all hospitalized polio cases were treated at St. Francis Hospital in Peoria. However, in that year, St. Joseph's Hospital established an isolation ward for polio victims, most of them children, in a nine county area, becoming one of only three downstate polio treatment centers.[69] The Marian Unit, established at St. Joseph's in 1954, continued to serve victims of polio and other crippling diseases long after the Salk and Sabin vaccines became available in the late 1950s.

In addition to care for certain categories of patients, in the mid-twentieth century hospitals began to offer formal facilities for emergency treatment. Before this time, accident victims and people suddenly taken acutely ill were dealt with informally. First aid was administered by whomever was first on the scene. Thus, policemen often dealt with victims of car accidents; funeral home directors ran ambulance services. For example, A.H. Otto of Danvers used a converted hearse as an ambulance beginning in 1925. In the 1940s, he charged 35¢ a mile, or about $3.85, for a trip to St. Joseph's Hospital.[70] Doctors either dealt with emergency patients in their homes or attended them at accident scenes, often transporting them to hospitals themselves. Emergency rooms and specialized ambulance services developed in the decades after World War II, although 24-hour coverage and trauma centers were not available locally until the 1970s.

The introduction of antibiotics to the civilian population after World War II heralded a revolution in hospital organization and care. Life-threatening infections which had kept patients in bed for weeks and months at a time could be dealt with in a matter of days. Hospital stays got shorter; hospital treatment became more specialized. The potential for surgery became virtually unlimited as concern about post-operative infection diminished. At the same time, development of an ever-expanding array of medical equipment converted hospitals into high-tech factories for the production of health.

Conclusions

The history of McLean County's hospitals is one of change and expansion. In just over a century, from relatively small facilities used by a tiny percentage of the population, the community's hospitals have become necessary major institutions, used by virtually all residents at various points in their lives. Hospitals are physical manifestations of the changes in health care delivery, reflecting specialization, technological innovation, and the institutionalization of care. They also reflect the social transformations of the twentieth century, altering from institutions which separated poor from rich, white from black, to institutions offering the same resources for the treatment of ill health regardless of the status of the sufferer.

Like American hospitals generally, McLean County's hospitals have also changed from charitable facilities operating on shoestring budgets to major business enterprises. Although still firmly grounded on the altruistic priciples of their founders, the County's hospitals have followed national trends in offering increasingly luxurious settings in which to suffer, accompanied by costs and charges which rise faster than the rate of inflation. Competition and collaboration have gone hand in hand as the hospitals have identified unique market niches or duplicated high-demand services.

In the next century, these hospitals face challenges every bit as daunting as those encountered during the last hundred years. As costs increase, occupancy rates fall. As health care occupations become increasingly skilled and professionalized, wages rise. Along with physicians and patients, hospitals are being challenged to adapt to new needs and demands. It is possible that hospitals may increasingly take on the role of managers, rather than locations, of care for members of their communities. Aspects of their own histories which looked very old-fashioned in 1950, such as dispensary and visiting nursing services, may become increasingly attractive in the near future. Whatever the changes, however, McLean County's hospitals will build them on the strength of a strong foundation of community service.

Case Study: St. Joseph's Hospital, 1880-1906

The work of the historian is often like that of a quilter, who patches together pieces collected from a variety of sources in order to make a finished product which hangs together. This study is such a patchwork. However, sometimes historians get lucky. This chapter is based on three primary sources regarding the first quarter century of St. Joseph's Hospital's existence: minutes of hospital staff meetings held between 1885 and 1902; hospital admissions records for the years from 1880 to 1906; and hospital accounts kept between 1880 and 1898. These sources create an intimate and detailed view of what life was like for the physicians, patients, and nursing sisters in a time very different from our own.

Doctors

When Reverend Mother Francis and Sister Augustine of St. Francis Hospital, Peoria, visited Bloomington in 1879 to explore the possibility of opening a new hospital, they discussed the project with two local physicians, Dr. Charles R. Parke (1823-1908) and Dr. John Sweeney (1840-1883). These doctors agreed to assemble a medical staff for St. Joseph's Hospital, which opened the following year.

Dr. Parke was then in his late fifties and had been practicing medicine in Bloomington for over thirty years. Having obtained his medical training at the University of Pennsylvania during the 1840s, Parke moved west to Whiteside County, Illinois, in 1848. This move was apparently not sufficient to slake his thirst for adventure; in 1849, Parke joined a company of gold-seekers and traveled to California. In the early '50s, he returned to Illinois *via* Central America, only to leave again, accepting a commission as a surgeon in the Russian army in 1855 during the Crimean War. When the war ended, Parke journeyed back to the United States by way of Berlin, Paris and London, augmenting his medical education in those European capitals. In 1857, he returned to Bloomington and established a practice which continued for nearly fifty years. Parke specialized in the diseases of the eye and ear and in general surgery.

Nearly a generation younger than Parke, Dr. John Sweeney received his formal medical education at Albany Medical College in New York at the "session of 1859 and 1860" — training much amplified by his experience as an Assistant Surgeon with the

Union army during the Civil War. He arrived in Normal in 1865, and became the first Medical Attendant of the Soldiers' Orphans' Home. He later became Dr. Parke's partner.[1]

St. Joseph's first medical staff included Doctors Parke and Sweeney, Dr. A.H. Luce (1816-1893), Dr. T.F. Worrell (1821-1887), Dr. William Elder (1826-1895), Dr. R. Wunderlich (1833-1893), and Dr. Lee Smith (1832-1911). Each doctor agreed "to serve without pay, except, of course, private patients whom they may recommend to the hospital for the superior nursing."[2] Together with four nursing sisters, led by their Superior, Sister Augustine, these physicians provided the medical care received by the 61 patients hospitalized at St. Joseph's in 1880.

The Waddle property, purchased by the Order for $7,000 to house the new hospital, was "an old brick mansion," located at the corner of Jackson Street and Morris Avenue at the center of a seven-acre tract of land. Although grand, the former private home was not ideal for hospital uses, and could accommodate only a few patients at a time. For example, only two patients were admitted in May, 1880; during most of that first year, fewer than four patients occupied beds at any given time. The addition of a purpose-built hospital building in 1883 expanded the hospital's capacity to 42 beds and made it possible for the old building to be used as a residence and chapel for the sisters. The nursing staff also expanded, by 1886 generally including approximately 12 sisters at any given time.

The hospital was run by the nuns, who, with the help of several hired men, grew and prepared most of the food consumed by patients and staff, kept the building clean, did the laundry, and cared for patients. Staff physicians made no administrative decisions, although they did make recommendations. While committed to the success of the hospital, their professional activities were largely performed outside its doors. The annual report for 1887 indicated that "one or more members of the medical staff visits the hospital daily."[3] However, these visits were generally made only to the physician's own patients, since the staff had agreed early on about the "necessity and propriety of patients keeping one physician for an attendant."[4]

The medical staff's primary involvement with hospital management during the 1880s and 1890s was to provide a Sanitary Inspector, whose regular reports on hospital facilities and needs provided the main topic for discussion at staff meetings which occurred monthly before 1887, and quarterly until the end of the record in 1902. The position rotated from one staff member to another. In November and December of 1885, for instance, Dr. A.T. Barnes (1832-1901) was Sanitary Inspector. At the November staff meeting:

> He reported the drug room, operating room, halls, wards, and private rooms, water closet, outhouses, etc., as in excellent condition. The patients are doing well and well pleased. He thought the wash room ought to be supplied with a steam washing machine and a mangle, and the kitchen with a steam table for vegetables that the sisters might be able to work to better advantage.

At the following month's meeting, Dr. Barnes recommended that the hospital purchase an elevator, a suggestion which was reiterated by Dr. William Elder (1826-1895) when he served as Sanitary Inspector in early 1886.[5] The Sanitary Inspector reported when the hospital was connected with the newly constructed city sewer system in May, 1886, and recommended the use of disinfectants in water closets.[6]

The physicians' sanitary inspection activities indicate the developing association between professional medicine and the germ theory of disease causation. Although the formal medical education received between 1840 and 1860 by St. Joseph's staff physicians could not have included laboratory training in microbiology, by the 1880s doctors, as medical experts, were expected to be able to recognize situations which could provide breeding grounds for microbes, and thus help to prevent the infections which persistently dogged nineteenth-century hospitals.

It is noteworthy that St. Joseph's staff physicians were somewhat defensive about deaths occurring in the hospital, ascribing unusually high mortality figures in 1890, 1891 and 1893 "to the septic condition of the atmosphere due to presence of 'grippe' [i.e., flu]. . . ." This comment indicates the extent to which physicians still clung to the miasma theory of disease causation. The physicians also explained deaths by saying that patients were often admitted to the hospital "in a dying condition, living only a few hours." In addition, they differentiated between preventable and inevitable deaths, in 1888 reporting:

> We have had only sixteen deaths during the last year out of 234 patients admitted, and of these, eight were necessarily fatal. Two with cancer, two old age, three phthisis pulmonalis [tuberculosis], and one a shoulder crushed under

the railroad cars, leaving only eight cases legitimate subjects for medical and surgical treatment, a little over 3 percent, which compares favorably with any hospital record.[7]

Low mortality was attributed to good hospital sanitation.
For example, the Sanitary Inspector found the hospital "in excellent sanitary condition" in October 1888, "notwithstanding the fact
that most of the time every bed has been occupied by patients, a
large proportion of whom have been surgical cases, [but] there has
not been a single case of hospital gangrene or erysipelas occurring
among them."[8]

In addition to the reports of the Sanitary Inspector, medical
staff meetings also provided a forum for discussion of physicians'
own needs regarding hospital facilities. In an era when most ailments were suffered and treated in patients' homes, hospitals
were considered useful for only a narrow range of activities. Chief
among these was surgery. In 1893, the medical staff discussed the
question of building a new operating room:

> It is the intention to supply the new room with a complete
> set of new and improved instruments supplemented by a
> fine operating table which, being constructed entirely of
> glass and iron, will leave no infection after being cleansed.
> The interior of the apartment will be conveniently arranged
> and the floor will probably be cemented. After being used,
> the instruments will be boiled and placed on a rack and
> kept so that contamination will be impossible. Everything
> that is possible according to the most approved methods
> will be done to contribute to the efficiency and safety of the
> room, and it is probable that when completed it will be
> equal in appointments to the best in the state.[9]

The room was constructed in 1895 according to the most up-
to-date principles of surgery. "To prevent septic poisoning the walls
were constructed of glass and steel, the floor of cement. Thorough
drainage was secured, and the rooms can be flooded with superheated steam, thus reducing the danger of sepsis to the minimum." The hospital paid $88.25 for the operating table and $325
to the carpenter.[10]

Medical staff members also occasionally made suggestions
regarding the nursing sisters' activities. For example, in 1891 one
physician asked the staff to recommend that the nuns use a blank
form for keeping consistent patient records "whereby cases could

be followed up from day to day." The Medical staff voted that the blanks "be placed before the sisters for their adoption."[11] In 1897, the staff indicated a need for additional sisters and recommended that sisters devote their time solely to nursing, rather than to other household tasks:

> With the increase of business we need new sisters, in order that the nurses proper shall not be required to do anything except care for their patients, thus enabling them to keep their hands and clothing in as perfectly an aseptic condition as possible.[12]

Records of medical staff meetings indicate the extent to which McLean County physicians were reconceptualizing the local practice of medicine to include hospitalization, and identifying the services hospitals could most usefully provide to the community. While several staff physicians had had experience in military and mental hospitals, none of them had been associated with a charitable general hospital. Thus, medical staff meetings occasionally considered the direction the hospital should take. Perhaps responding to the negative image clinging to nineteenth century hospitals, Dr. Parke observed in 1888 that "the character of the hospital itself has gradually changed from that of a general public hospital to that of a sanitary home for the sick and invalids." Physicians took pride in St. Joseph's appearance, themselves donating trees to be planted on hospital grounds, and praised the hospital's comfort and interior decoration, claiming in 1887, "There is not a room in the building which any citizen of Bloomington could not occupy with comfort and satisfaction. . . ."[13]

What kinds of conditions should be treated in the local hospital? While there was general agreement about surgical cases, there was some controversy about patients suffering from emotional illnesses. In 1895 the physicians discussed "the propriety of receiving insane patients into the hospital." Although admissions records indicate that the emotionally ill were routinely treated at St. Joseph's, the medical staff decided at that time that it was "not for the best interest of other patients that insane persons should be admitted."[14] Nonetheless, sufficient local need existed for Dr. Parke in 1898 to call for construction of "a detached building fitted up specially for patients suffering from mental disease."[15]

Although McLean County never built a facility for mental patients, there was clearly a need for institutional care for local sufferers. As we have seen, both St. Joseph's medical staff and the governing board of the Poor Farm considered constructing separate housing for the insane.[16] Furthermore, despite the doctors' general objections, St. Joseph's regularly admitted patients suffering from ailments including "monomania", "acute mania," "nervousness", "neurosis", and "insanity".[17] In the twentieth century, McLean County's emotionally ill were routinely sent to the mental hospital at Bartonville.

In addition to other emotional illnesses, the hospital often accommodated sufferers from "alcoholism"; 3.5 percent of admissions between 1880 and 1906 for which diagnosis was noted were victims of this disorder. There is some evidence that for many years St. Joseph's served as the drunk tank for Bloomington-Normal, housing the inebriated in rooms in the basement which, "although not as handsomely furnished as those on the other three floors, . . . are very comfortable and may be used in a case of necessity."[18] The sufferer was generally ready for discharge within 14 days.

Thus, despite their lack of interest in treating non-physical ailments, St. Joseph's staff physicians were regularly called upon to deal with mental disorders. That they and the nursing sisters undertook this apparently onerous responsibility indicates their dedication to community service. The charitable community hospital was designed to meet the general health care needs of residents — needs which were mental and spiritual as well as physical.

Patients

What do we know about the people who were admitted to St. Joseph's Hospital during the first quarter century of its existence? Between 1880 and 1906, 4,695 patients were accommodated. Gender was not indicated for 5 percent of admissions; of the remainder, 41 percent were female and 54 percent were male. Patients' ages ranged from two weeks to 95 years. However, very few children were admitted; indeed, only 3 percent of admissions were of people under age ten. The mean age of patients in this period was 41, with the largest concentrations being of people in their twenties and those over age 61.

St. Joseph's was, of course, a Catholic hospital, established by German nuns. Thus, it is not surprising that large numbers of patients were Catholic and foreign born. Indeed, one expert explains the dramatic growth in the number of Catholic hospitals in the late nineteenth century as "a consequence not simply of the specific history and commitment of the church and its religious orders, but of the isolated and defensive character of the Catholic immigrant population in American cities."[19] The first white settlers in McLean County were of Yankee Protestant stock. Catholic Irish and Germans were relative newcomers lacking, in many cases, the resources to support medical treatment within their own homes. These were the people Sister Augustine and her companion sisters came to Bloomington to serve.

Nonetheless, as the only hospital in the community for over a decade, St. Joseph's admitted patients with a wide range of ethnic and religious backgrounds. Of those early patients indicating religious affiliation, 44 percent were Catholic and 21 percent were Protestant. Many were immigrants. Despite the fact that only 13 percent of McLean County's residents were foreign born in 1880, only 40 percent of patients appearing in the admissions records were born in the United States. Three out of ten were Irish and one sixth were German. The hospital also admitted English, Swedish, French, Polish, Chinese, Belgian, Scottish, Danish, Canadian, Italian, Bohemian, Syrian and Welsh patients. St. Joseph's also admitted at least 35 African American patients during the period under consideration.[20]

St. Joseph's was established as a charitable hospital with a mission to serve sufferers regardless of their ability to pay for treatment. In fact, from the beginning, most patients paid something toward the cost of their treatment, an amount presumably calculated according to their financial resources. The treatment of some was paid for by the County at a negotiated rate which increased as time went on.[21] Only a few patients, identified by Dr. Parke as "those who had neither home, money or friends", were treated free of charge.[22] The proportion of patients in this category ranged from less than one percent in some years to eight percent of the total number of patients treated in 1900.

The amount paid for hospital care ranged from one to five hundred dollars. Larger amounts were paid for "a home for life" than for any medical service. The median amount paid was five dollars, regardless of the treatment rendered or the duration of stay. However, in the years between 1880 and 1906, the average charge for hospital care increased (see Table 1).

Table 1: Payment for Hospital Care

Year	Amount most patients paid
1880	$3.00
1881-1895	$5.00
1899	$7.00
1903-1905	$10.00

Most of the money paid by patients was for "board": very little went toward other expenses, such as medicine.[23]

A wide range of health problems brought patients to St. Joseph's Hospital in the period under consideration. Diagnoses were not recorded for 65 percent of people admitted. For the remainder, which includes 1,438 cases, recorded diagnoses were considered within 22 broad categories, of which six occurred most frequently: miscellaneous surgeries, fevers, injuries, alcoholism, contagious diseases and miscellaneous ailments (see Table 2).[24]

Table 2: Diagnoses of patients admitted to St. Joseph's Hospital, 1880-1906

Diagnosis	Percent of patients
Miscellaneous	7.4
Alcoholism	3.5
Injury (excluding fractures)	3.1
Misc. surgeries	2.7
Misc. contagious diseases	2.7
Misc. fevers	2.2
Joint, back & nerves	1.6
Mental illness	1.5
Local infections	1.5
Respiratory (excluding t.b.)	1.3
Tuberculosis	1.3
Gastrointestinal problems	1.2
Dropsy	.8
Fractures	.7
Heart problems	.7
Cancers	.6
Amputations	.5
Boarding (e.g., living in hospital)	.4
Poisoning	.4
Epilepsy	.1

Worthy of note are the conditions *not* appearing on this list. For example, the hospital delivered fewer than five babies during the entire study period. No tonsillectomies were performed. The only cancers treated were of the breast and uterus. It is also noteworthy, however, that the hospital dealt with conditions which are rarely or never seen in McLean County today, including malaria, smallpox, and erysipelas.

The first patient treated at St. Joseph's hospital was Mrs. Rosie Flanagan, a 45-year old Catholic Irishwoman from Bloomington, admitted on March 22, 1880, with a diagnosis of breast cancer. Dr. Parke removed the tumor and the patient was discharged two weeks later, "recovered."

Most of the patients treated at St. Joseph's during the period under consideration were discharged as recovered (46%) or improved (12%). A significant percentage (7.1%) were classified as having "left" the hospital, either without being officially discharged, or without change in their condition. A small number of patients were discharged as incurable (2.3%). Only 479 of the 3,683 patients for whom outcomes are known died at St. Joseph's.

Not all of the "patients" accommodated at St. Joseph's Hospital were suffering from ill-health. For instance, on January 9, 1900, nine-year-old Jim Dolan and his two-year-old brother, Archie, were admitted with the diagnosis "Orphans". These Irish children stayed at the hospital for 181 days — presumably, until other accommodation could be found for them. In addition, a number of elderly patients purchased a home for life at St. Joseph's.

How long did patients stay in the hospital during this period? Length of stay varied greatly, ranging from one to 1,821 days, and depended upon factors including diagnosis and the age of the patient. Chronic physical and mental disorders (with the exception of alcoholism) were associated with comparatively longer hospital stays, as was general debility and old age. Conversely, a majority of the patients suffering from alcoholism, injuries, conditions requiring surgery, fevers, and gastrointestinal ailments were discharged in less than fourteen days. Generally speaking, hospital stays were long. In 1891, the average stay lasted for 52 days.[25]

What was a hospital stay like in this period? Hospitals offered few private rooms and no private baths. While accommodations were more luxurious than those of many private homes of the period, they were spartan compared to those provided by modern hospitals. Rooms were simple bedrooms, generally without any specialized hospital equipment. Patients came to the hospital for nursing care, which was St. Joseph's specialty and its pride.

Both illness and convalescence lasted longer at the turn of the century than they do today. Thus, once the acute period of suffering had passed, patients enjoyed the use of the hospital's grounds. In 1890, Dr. Parke wrote:

Large trees in great abundance afford shade and shelter.

In the summer time the beautiful lawns, decorated with flowers and laid out by walks; the sisters dressed in their black and white garments walking hither and thither, followed by a faithful dog; here and there sitting at the foot of some tree patients sufficiently recovered to be out in the open air; the singing of the birds and the quiet that reigns about the neighborhood all remind one of those ideal refuges pictured in story books.[26]

Patients also occasionally took part in social occasions organized by the hospital. After the annual meeting in 1894, there was a party during which:

Father Donavan, a well known former clergyman of this city, who is now a patient at the hospital, and Dr. Godfrey gave a violin duet, assisted by Miss Mayme Schell, who is also a patient. The gentlemen are talented players, and the trio gave a charming concert. Mrs. Dr. G.R. Smith, who has an excellent voice, sang several selections sweetly. Dr. Corley also sang a solo.[27]

Thus, long-term patients had a far different relationship with hospital staff members than is usual a century later.

Nurses and Hospital Management

Very little is known about the nursing sisters who established and ran St. Joseph's hospital during its first quarter century of existence. Having emigrated from Germany as a result of Otto von Bismarck's anti-Catholic policies, they offered the expertise garnered in the military hospitals of the Franco-Prussian War (1870-1) to residents of the American midwest. Having been assigned to their Order's hospitals in Peoria, Bloomington and, eventually, other locations, their individual identities were absorbed in the endless work of growing, harvesting and preparing food for hospital staff and patients; keeping buildings and laundry clean; managing hospital finances and records; and providing 24-hour nursing care to patients. As nuns, they lived apart from the community they served. Yet, glimpses of their lives and special talents are offered in the hospital records.

The nuns were involved in all hospital activities and projects. For example, in 1887 the Sanitary Inspector reported:

Since our last report of a month ago, the sisters, especially Sister Ludovica, aided by Mr. Rothmann, teacher in the German school, have painted and frescoed all the wards and nearly all the departments of the hospital in a style that would do credit to our best painters.[28]

Other useful talents included fund-raising. The sisters collected money for the hospital from individuals and businesses, including the local coal mine, which was a generous and regular donor. They also ran raffles.[29]

The hospital was located in the midst of "several acres of rich, high land upon which is raised nearly all the vegetables used in the institution."[30] With the help of several hired men, paid between $18 and $25 per month, the nuns farmed this land, subcontracting only the ploughing. They also took care of the hospital's livestock, which generally included a cow, several horses and chickens. The purchase and care of these animals represented a major expense for the new hospital. For instance, in February of 1889, when the hospital accounts showed a balance of only $727.33, the sisters paid a total of $47.50 for a new cow. Horseshoes, feed, and occasional veterinarian bills were comparatively expensive. However, animals were also valuable investments. In December 1885, the sisters were paid $186 "for our little horse."

In addition to other tasks, the nuns also managed the hospital's finances. It is noteworthy how little money changed hands in early days. For example, during April 1880, the hospital received $168.35 and spent $174.52. Income came from patients' fees, charitable donations and contributions from the Order. Expenditures were for medicine, shoes, dry goods, animal feed, groceries which could not be grown on the property (including regular payments for oysters!), labor done by workmen, utilities, travel by the sisters to collect money and visit the Mother House in Peoria, and building projects. Throughout the period covered by the record, between March 1880 and June 1898, both income and day-to-day expenses were very small by today's standards. The only large sums mentioned are the amounts borrowed for building projects. For example, in January 1888, St. Joseph's owed $4,000 to the Mercantile National Bank, $2,000 to Mr. Fred Ruppenkamp, $1,160 to Rev. B. Baak and $615 to Mrs. Sarah Adams. Aside from this debt, its cash balance was $443.57.[31]

Despite these small amounts and the shoestring budget on which the hospital operated, the sisters managed to serve a great many people. January of 1888 provides a useful example. (Januaries were always busy at St. Joseph's.) In that month, 35 patients were admitted to an already full facility. Most of these people stayed more than one month; only three left within two weeks. No one paid more than $7 for his or her accommodation. In January 1888, the sisters collected $420.76 from patients and spent $442.57. While the hospital did not always operate at a loss, it took all the sisters' intelligence and hard work to keep it a going concern. It was also significant that the nuns worked without monetary payment. As Dr. Parke wrote of them in 1887, "The sisters of this order only expect a living in this world, the proceeds of their labor being expended in increasing their facilities for doing good."[32]

Caring For Strangers: Nurse Training and Nursing

The face of Mrs. Gamp — the nose in particular — was somewhat red and swollen, and it was difficult to enjoy her society without becoming conscious of a smell of spirits. Like most persons who have attained to great eminence in their profession, she took to hers very kindly; insomuch that, setting aside her natural predilections as a woman, she went to a lying-in or a laying-out with equal zest and relish.

Charles Dickens, <u>Martin Chuzzlewit</u>, (1843-4)

The Image of the Nurse

Nursing has always been considered to be an integral part of a good woman's role. In most times, places and cultures, wives, mothers and neighbors have nurtured and cared for the sick. Self-sacrifice, sympathy and empathy are at the heart of traditional ideas about "natural" femininity. However, nursing was only respectable when it was unpaid. In Europe and North America before the late nineteenth century, paid nurses were of low status and had bad reputations. Employed by hospitals or hired on a temporary casual basis to work in private homes, they were drawn from the lowest social classes. Paid very little, valued less, nurses dealt with the messes and miseries that servants refused to handle. Although Charles Dickens's Sairey Gamp was a caricature, she would have been recognized as typical by mid-nineteenth-century readers.

From Sairey Gamp to the Lady with the Lamp, the image of the nurse changed dramatically in the second half of the nineteenth century. In contrast to its traditional association with ignorance, poverty, dirt and vice, nursing was increasingly linked to absolute cleanliness, skilled expertise and personal refinement. In the United States, this transformation began during the Civil War, when middle- and upper-class women became involved in nursing as a patriotic service they could render to the men at the front lines. Following the example set by Florence Nightingale in the British military hospitals of the Crimean War a decade earlier, American nursing reformers sought to bring order and good management to hospital nursing. As a result of their recognition of the dismal lack of skill among the volunteers staffing wartime military hospitals, the first American nursing schools organized on the Nightingale model were established during the 1870s.[1]

This development had far-ranging effects. It created an opportunity for a respectable career outside the home for middle-class American women. It helped to change the image of the hospital from a place of disorder, filth, infection and death to an orderly sanctuary for sufferers filled with fresh air, nourishing food and clean sheets. It also transformed the staffing, structure and finances of American hospitals. Early on, hospital boards and administrators realized that a nursing school could supply a hospital with an inexhaustible supply of young, strong, biddable, and at least partially trained labor at a fraction of the wages demanded by either untrained servants or graduate nurses. Thus, by 1923 one quarter of the 6,830 hospitals in the United States had their own nursing schools.

Early nursing schools emphasized discipline, character and technical competence. Within the hospital's hierarchical network, the student nurse was superior only to hospital servants, but inferior to graduate nurse supervisors, nursing superintendants, physicians and board members. Obedience and deference were required, independent judgement discouraged. Student nurses were expected to develop personal characters which combined self sacrifice with dignity and morality. Demeanor was very important; a student nurse must act like a lady. She was discouraged from using slang, getting involved in pranks, or becoming too familiar with domestic servants or patients. Pregnancy or drunkenness usually resulted in expulsion. Competence in the few technical skills required of nineteenth-century nurses was inculcated by repeating procedures until they became automatic. According to Isabel Hampton Robb, nursing superintendant at Johns Hopkins Hospital in Baltimore, "There is a right way and that is the one and only one she must learn. Only by constant repetition can you become really familiar with the work."[2]

Nurse training emphasized work rather than academic preparation. Although they attended lectures, usually given by the hospital's medical staff, student nurses were expected to devote between ten and thirteen hours a day, six days a week, to the day-to-day work of the hospital. One expert describes student nurses in the period before about 1920 as "an army of mechanical women bent on incessant cleaning."[3] Although the image of the nurse had changed, the nature of the work required of nurses remained the same as it had been in the early nineteenth century.

Nursing was hard and unremitting labor. The following instructions and advice given to floor nurses at Cleveland Lutheran Hospital in 1887 illustrate the working conditions of nurses at that time:

> In addition to caring for your 50 patients, each nurse will follow these regulations:
> 1. Daily sweep and mob the floors of your ward, dust the patient's furniture and window sills.
> 2. Maintain an even temperature in your ward by bringing in a scuttle of coal for the day's business.
> 3. Light is important to observe the patient's condition. Therefore, each day fill kerosene lamps, clean chimneys, and trim wicks. Wash windows once a week.
> 4. The nurse's notes are important in aiding the physician's work. Make your pens carefully. You may whittle nibs to your individual taste.
> 5. Each nurse on duty will report every day at 7 a.m. and leave at 8 p.m. except on the Sabbath on which you will be off from 12 noon to 2 p.m..
> 6. Graduate nurses in good standing with the Director of Nurses will be given an evening off each week for courting purposes, or two evenings a week if you go to church regularly.
> 7. Each nurse should lay aside from each pay a goodly sum of her earnings for her benefits during her declining years, so that she will not become a burden. For example, if you earn $30 a month you should set aside $15.
> 8. Any nurse who smokes, uses liquor in any form, gets her hair done at a beauty shop, or frequents dance halls will give the Director of Nurses good reason to suspect her intentions, worth and integrity.
> 9. The nurse who performs her labor, serves her patients and doctors faithfully and without fault for a period of five years will be given an increase by the hospital administration of 5 cents a day providing there are no hospital debts that are outstanding.[4]

In hospitals with training schools, student nurses did most of the patient care and housework. In return, they received room and board and, after a probationary period, a monthly allowance or stipend of between eight and twelve dollars. Hospitals also collected fees when students did special or private duty nursing.

Before the mid-twentieth century, there were no standardized entrance requirements or curriculum for nursing schools. Applicants for nurse training were expected to be of good character and in sturdy physical health. Both character and health were tested during the customary two-year training period.

Despite the hospitals' exploitation of student labor and the imbalance between work and study, nursing became an increasingly popular career opportunity for young women. While not, perhaps, as high status a job as teaching, nursing was considered less menial than factory work or domestic service. The supervision and regimentation of nurse training appealed to parents. In a nation where more than half the population lived in rural settlements, nursing school offered a protected opportunity to experience urban life. Thus, for many young women, nursing became an attractive route to financial and social independence.

Nursing Careers

Despite the proliferation of nursing schools, there were no standardized requirements for graduation or licenses for practice. Because the schools were owned and operated by hospitals, the hospital's need for labor took priority over the student nurse's need for training. The quality and extent of graduate nurses' skills varied greatly from one school to another. In the 1890s, a group of nursing superintendants began to advocate formation of professional nursing organizations to improve the quality of nursing education and regulate the practice of nursing. The establishment of the Nurses' Associated Alumnae Association (NAAA) of the United States and Canada (later renamed the American Nurses' Association) in 1897 provided a forum and a vehicle for professionalization.[5]

At about the same time, state organizations were developing. The Illinois Graduate Nurse's Association was founded in 1901 with the primary goal of bringing about state registration of nurses.[6] In 1911, this association reorganized on the basis of geographical districts associated with railroad facilities. In 1914, the 6th District of the Illinois State Association of Graduate Nurses, which then included McLean, Livingston (except for the town of Dwight), Ford, DeWitt and Logan counties, was established. The following year, the district expanded to include Kankakee and Iroquois counties. Students graduating from nursing schools in this region joined both district and state organizations, thus

118

becoming registered nurses. This network helped to both standardize and regulate nursing in Illinois. Because of the close relationship between nursing schools and hospitals, nurses who were not members of alumnae associations would have found it very difficult to get work, either on hospital staffs or as private duty nurses.

The efforts of professional organizations were supported in 1923 by publication of the Goldmark Report, which many hoped would have the same impact on nursing that the Flexner Report of 1910 had had on medicine. The Goldmark Report, commissioned by the Rockefeller Foundation, considered the contemporary condition of nursing education and made recommendations for the future of professional nursing. It called for:

> the maintenance of high educational standards, including
> more basic science courses; a properly funded training
> school with a graded curriculum of twenty-eight months;
> and the endowment of a university-based school of nursing
> to train the profession's future leadership. Further, in a
> fairly controversial section, it called for the replacement of
> student nurses by graduates in hospitals and the training
> of "hospital helpers" in the execution of routine duties of a
> "non-educational character."[7]

Although the report received a mixed reception when it came out, it was prophetic about the direction nursing would take during the next half-century.

Before about 1940, most graduate nurses did private duty nursing, either in hospitals or in patients' homes. Hospitals managed "registers" which assigned private duty jobs to nurses on a rotating basis. In addition, physicians often called upon their favorite nurses to care for their own patients. Private duty, though demanding, was reasonably lucrative. However, within the profession, this work conferred lower status than the relatively few hospital staff positions. Furthermore, as the need for long-term private duty nursing decreased in the twentieth century, both the status of and the market for private duty nurses declined. During the lean years of the Depression, graduate nurses were chronically underemployed. Only the development in the 1940s of the new demand on the part of hospitals for qualified nurses eased this situation. With the introduction of intensive care wards in hospitals after World War II, the private duty nurse virtually disappeared.

As patient populations and the demand for specialized

nursing skills grew in the mid-twentieth century, hospitals began to employ growing numbers of graduate nurses. The parallel trend in nursing education away from on-the-job training and towards academic preparation reduced the amount of time student nurses could devote to hospital work. Hospital staffs grew and became increasingly diversified. After World War II, nurses did not wash floors or clean bathrooms. However, they *did* insert I.V.s and assist with increasingly complicated and ambitious surgical procedures. They also helped complete the growing range of paperwork required by the developing relationship between hospitals, physicians and insurance companies. Nurses' responsibilities required increasingly advanced educations. Thus, graduate nurses became the backbone of hospital staffs, and hospitals stopped depending upon student labor.

In the second half of the twentieth century, the time student nurses spent on hospital wards was considered educational experience, rather than a contribution to the work necessary to run the hospital. It is noteworthy that they were no longer paid stipends; rather, their student status was both indicated and protected by their payment of tuition. Nursing schools became functionally distinct from hospitals, often associating with universities to offer high quality theoretical and laboratory training as well as the option of a bachelor's degree.

McLean County's Nursing Schools

All of McLean County's major hospitals had nurse training schools. The Kelso Sanitarium and Mennonite Hospital began training nurses when they opened in 1894 and 1920 respectively.[8] From the beginning, these hospitals followed the nationally typical model of employing graduate nurses as superintendents and department supervisors, but using student labor for most of the patient care and housekeeping.

St. Joseph's and Deaconess (later Brokaw) hospitals initially depended upon the efforts of spiritually committed nuns and deaconesses who worked without pay for the love of God and their keep. For Deaconess Hospital, this arrangement was unsuccessful. First Mennonite, then Methodist deaconesses provided nursing services in the years immediately following the hospital's establishment in 1896. However, the deaconesses were not as well trained, biddable or plentiful as student nurses would be. By the turn of the century, Deaconess Hospital was training nurses and depending upon student labor.[9]

With the organizational and human resources of the Sisters of the Third Order of St. Francis behind it, St. Joseph's Hospital had less need of student labor than other McLean County hospitals. However, in 1920, the hospital opened its third major addition, greatly increasing the number of patients it could accommodate at any one time. Its needs having outgrown the capacity of the Order to supply nurses, St. Joseph's Hospital opened a School of Nursing in 1921. This school operated until 1962, when St. Joseph's was employing increasing numbers of graduate nurses.

The histories of the nursing schools run by Brokaw and Mennonite hospitals illustrate typical, but contrasting, developments occurring in American nursing education during the twentieth century. Both schools extended their programs from two to three years in length — Brokaw in the early 1920s and Mennonite in the 1940s. However, perhaps in response to the Goldmark Report, Brokaw affiliated with Illinois Wesleyan University in 1923 to provide students with the option of receiving a bachelor of science degree at the same time as becoming a graduate nurse. Plans for the formation of a fully collegiate school of nursing continued. In 1956, Brokaw's program changed its name to Brokaw Hospital School for Nursing of Illinois Wesleyan University. In 1962, this school graduated its last class, and Illinois Weslyan University opened its own nursing program.[10]

In contrast to Brokaw's early development of a degree program, Mennonite Hospital's School of Nursing remained committed to the three-year diploma long after degree programs had become the usual form of preparation for nursing careers. Although the academic component of its curriculum was strengthened to include course work at Illinois State Normal University (ISNU) in 1945, until the late 1960s Mennonite's nursing school "was an apprenticeship style of training based on a strong learning-by-doing philosophy."[11] During the 1970s, the curriculum was augmented by both additional theoretical course work and a variety of experiential placements for students. In 1982, the Mennonite College of Nursing was established, offering a baccalaureate curriculum enhanced by partnerships with seven Illinois institutions of higher education.

The Experience of Nurse Training

This study benefits enormously from oral history interviews conducted with eight nurses born between 1909 and 1938. The oldest respondent, Ruth Carpenter, began her training at

Brokaw's Nursing School in 1928. The youngest, Sally Wagner, participated in the diploma program at Grant Hospital, Chicago, in the late 1950s. Sister Theonilla, born in 1912, was the only interviewee to attend a two-year nurse training program. Five respondents participated in three-year diploma programs. Evelyn Lantz, born in 1918, received a scholarship in 1935 to attend the five-year degree course jointly offered by Brokaw Nursing School and Illinois Wesleyan University. Three respondents earned Bachelor's degrees; one went on to get a Master's in nursing.

Table 1: Nurses

Respondent	Birthdate	Nursing school(s)	Qualification
Ruth Carpenter	1909	Brokaw Nursing School	Diploma
Sister Theonilla	1912	Keokuk, Iowa	Diploma
Evelyn Lantz	1918	Brokaw/Illinois Wesleyan	B.S.
Roberta Holman	1921	Brokaw Nursing School	Diploma
Sister Judith	1922	Düsseldorf, Germany	Diploma
Jane Tinsley	1924	Brokaw Nursing School	Diploma
Alice Swift	1927	Lancaster, PA	Diploma
		Eastern Mennonite College	B.S.
		Washington University	M.S.
Sally Wagner	1938	Grant Hospital, Chicago	Diploma

During the period covered by this study, there were tremendous changes in the expectations of and prerequisites for nurse training; the experience of nursing education; and the prospects facing graduate nurses. The oral history interviews lend a human face to the information provided by official histories and newspaper accounts.

Career Choice

Why did young women want to be nurses? The answer to this question varies depending upon individual personality and circumstances. For some respondents, nursing was a dramatic, heroic career. Others followed admired role models into the profession. For still others, nursing was a practical career choice — the best opportunity available.

Roberta Holman was attracted to nursing because of the profession's romantic image. She remembered,

> It was a dream thing. . . . I wanted to be a nurse when I was ten years old. I thought being a nurse just sounded wonderful. And then when I had occasion to visit people in the hospital. . . , I'd see these nurses walking down the hall

in these beautiful, white, starched uniforms and ah — that must be wonderful! You know! I wanted to wear one of those white uniforms.[12]

Her father and the high school superintendent discouraged her from undertaking nurse training, "because I was really skinny. I was the skinniest thing you'd ever seen. . . . They just thought that physically I could not handle it."[13] Despite his initial concern, Roberta's father was very proud of Roberta when she became a nurse. And, despite her size and the physical demands of her training course, Roberta never regretted her decision.

Jane Tinsley also became a nurse because of a childhood fantasy. She said, "I think I thought I was going to be by somebody's bedside in a little white uniform just taking care of them, making them well. It was the only thing I ever wanted to do. I never even thought about anything else."[14]

Ruth Carpenter followed a friend she admired into nursing. She grew up on a farm in Vermilion County, Illinois. Her mother died after giving birth to her brother when Ruth was four. Thereafter, Ruth spent several years in the Cunningham Children's Home in Champaign before her father remarried. At the Children's Home, Ruth's closest friend was a girl several years older than herself who became a nurse. This young woman inspired Ruth's interest in the profession. Ruth's father was unenthusiastic about her ambition, "because in those days nurses were pretty low on the totem pole as far as respectability is concerned. . . . In the early '20s . . . a lot of nurses were just not respectable."[15] His attitude reflected the much earlier association of nursing with vice. Nonetheless, Ruth stuck with her childhood ambition and after a year of studying to be a teacher at Illinois State Normal University (ISNU), she enrolled in Brokaw School of Nursing in 1928.

For Sister Theonilla of the Sisters of the Third Order of St. Francis, the decision to become a nurse was part of her religious vocation. Born and raised in Dortmund, Germany, her father was a skilled factory worker and her mother was a seamstress. She finished the standard eight years of education, then looked after her father's household for two years after her mother's death. Her aunt was a member of the religious order she eventually joined. Discussions with that family member influenced Sister Theonilla's decision to enter the convent at age 19 and to become a nurse. Previously, she had had no career ambitions and "never thought about getting married." Her decision to begin nurse training "was

made for me. You didn't make your own decisions in those days."
Sister Theonilla was sent to the Order's nursing school in Keokuk,
Iowa, to participate in a two-year diploma course which also
trained lay nurses.

In contrast to Sister Theonilla's experience, Sister Judith's
interest in nursing pre-dated her religious vocation, although she
had had a childhood interest in being a missionary. Born in
Dusseldorf, Germany, she began her nurse training in 1942 during
World War II. When asked what influenced her decision to become
a nurse, Sister Judith answered:

> I saw the work. One time I was in the emergency room and
> I saw the work they were doing to help people, so I decided
> I would like to work as a nurse to help people. These were
> compassionate and helping people. I think this was the
> reason for doing this.[16]

After the war ended, Sister Judith entered the convent and
applied to serve in the United States.

Like Sister Judith, Evelyn Lantz became interested in
nursing because of childhood exposure to the work:

> My grandfather Garner developed diabetes and he was in
> the hospital in Quincy. . . . My mother would take me with
> her to visit her father, my grandfather, in the hospital. I
> was about three years old. There were no rules or regula-
> tions about children being in the hospital. I was sort of a
> pet of the nurses and they would let me follow them
> around. I would sort of just tag along and I became very
> interested in what was going on in the examining rooms
> when they were cleaning them. Not when patients were in
> there, but when they would clean them, and just up and
> down the hall and that kind of thing. As I grew older, then
> I played nurse, you know, with a red cross on your head, or
> a dishrag to sort of wrap around your head or something or
> other to look like a nurse's cap.[17]

She was also attracted by the status and demeanor of nurses.
"Their families were respected families. They always seemed to be
very much in control and, how shall I say it, dignified. . . it wasn't
that they were reserved or anything of that kind, but very much in
command of the situation."[18]

Alice Swift's decision to become a nurse was based on a

practical assessment of the opportunities available to her. Born to an Amish Mennonite family in Iowa, Alice grew up in a very conservative religious community which viewed marriage and housework as the appropriate destiny for all young women. Members of the community "really opposed higher education, anything beyond elementary education." However, Alice liked to study and thought it was unlikely that she would marry young, since "somehow I never had dates." She said, "I did not look forward with anticipation and pleasure to the thought of doing housework the rest of my life if I wasn't going to get married." She persuaded her parents to send her to, first, a Mennonite high school in Virginia and then to a nursing school in Lancaster, Pennsylvania. This decision was unpopular with members of her community, among whom "professional nursing was seen as too much education." However, her parents supported her decision because "they had some rather liberal attitudes in a sense, so they didn't really create a big ruckus about my going."[19] Alice went on to take both a Bachelor's degree and a Master's in nursing.

Training

In 1921, the Brokaw Hospital School for Nurses advertised that it:

> offers to women desirious [sic] of becoming professional nurses, a course of practical and theoretical instruction. The practical knowledge is gained by actual care of patients, under the supervision of the Superintendent and her assistants. The theoretical course is of the best. The lecture corps, composed of members of the hospital staff, gives weekly lectures and daily clinical instruction. Classes in text-books are conducted by the Superintendent and her assistants.... Each student is given many opportunities for the special nursing of private patients, a work especially fitting her for duty as a graduate nurse.[20]

Applications were accepted at any time of year. Applicants were required to have finished at least one year of high school and to be between the ages of twenty and thirty-five. In addition to completing a one-page form providing biographical and health information, the aspiring nurse was asked to submit "a testimonial of character from her pastor or some clergyman who has known her at least five years, also a physician's certificate of health."

Students accepted to the program served a probationary

period of three months which could "in doubtful cases" be extended. During this time, students received board, lodging and laundry services. They were expected to bring with them to the school:

> Three wash dresses simply made, six large white aprons, several plain white collars, two bags for soiled linen, and a good supply of plain underclothing. Each article must be distinctly marked with owner's name in full. Each nurse will be required to have her own watch, also to wear rubber heeled shoes. If teeth are out of order, they should receive the necessary attention before entering.[21]

Once formally accepted as a pupil, the student nurse was allowed to wear the school's uniform, consisting "of a blue and white seersucker dress, white apron, cuffs, collar and cap." Students were expected to make their own uniforms of material supplied by the school. Students paid no tuition. In fact, after the probationary period, first-year pupils were paid monthly stipends of $8; second year students received $12 per month and third-year students were paid $15 per month. The school also provided textbooks.

The curriculum was organized into Junior (first-year), Intermediate, and Senior courses. In theory, course work was evenly divided between "practical" and "class and lecture" work.

Table 2: "Class and Lecture Work", Brokaw Hospital School for Nurses, 1921

Junior Course	Intermediate Course	Senior Course
Primary Anatomy	Preparation and after care of major surgical and obstetrical patients	Surgical and Medical Emergencies
Physiology and Hygiene	Bacteriology	Care of Children
Materia Medica	Surgical and Operating Room Technique	Contagious and Nervous Patients
Practical Nursing, including the entire care of ordinary medical, surgical and gynecological patients	General Medicine, Eye, Ear, Nose and Throat	Massage and Electricity
Urinalysis	Dietetics, theoretical and practical	Instruction by the Superintendent on Private Nursing Supplies
Cost and care of hospital supplies		Hygiene and Isolation in private homes

In practice, classroom education and study time were sandwiched in, when possible, between ward duties. Students worked long hours: day nurses, from 7 a.m. to 7 p.m.; night nurses from 7 p.m. to 7 a.m. They had little time off: "Pupils are allowed one-half day each week and one-half of Sunday."[22]

The professionalization of nursing was reflected in nurses' uniforms. Specific details of uniforms and caps indicated nursing students' progress and were matters of great pride. When Ruth Carpenter began her training at Brokaw Hospital in 1928,

> We had to make our own uniforms, which [were]... blue and white chambray with a belt and a full skirt. ... Of course, they gave you the apron and you wore that for six months and then you got your bib and cap and that sort of thing. And then they had white cuffs. We got the cuffs that were detachable. ... And sometimes we got to wear white shoes. Well, we got lazy and ... our white shoes didn't get so white. Then we had to wear black shoes and black stockings and, oh, that was awful. Those old black stockings and black shoes. ...[23]

By the time Evelyn Lantz went to Brokaw Hospital Nursing School in 1936, uniforms were provided. She described the changes in her uniform from entrance to "capping":

> I think it was three months that we were considered probation nurses. We didn't have the bib and the cap. Our uniform [was] chambray blue and white stripe, princess style with the white starched collar that you had to pin on and cuffs that had to be pinned on. After you passed your probationary period, you were given a cap, the cap of the school and a bib to go over your shoulders and cover the front of your uniform.[24]

Uniforms and caps remained important in nursing after World War II. Sally Wagner graduated from nursing school in 1959. She remembers a uniform similar to those worn twenty years before:

> When we went in ... our uniforms just consisted of a striped dres and a little pinafore. And then, when we had been there ... six months, they had a capping ceremony where you received your cap. And then, when you were a junior you got a stripe on your cap, and then ... when you were a senior I think the stripe came off, but you got a pin or something different. Then when you graduated you had your nursing pin and they had the graduation ceremony.[25]

Nurses were expected to keep their uniforms clean and tidy. They were also expected to learn how to clean hospital buildings and equipment according to nursing superintendents' exacting standards. Indeed, all respondents trained in diploma programs before World War II recall that their introduction to nursing school involved scrubbing. When Ruth Carpenter began her training in 1928,

> The first place I went to for any kind of service was in surgery. And we were taught to scrub anything that didn't move and some things that did move. We scrubbed everything. Surgical instruments and the floors and the woodwork and [everything with] soap and water.[26]

Eleven years later, Roberta Holman was introduced to nursing at Brokaw in the same way:

> Back then the first thing you learned was cleanliness. If you didn't know it you learned it then. They had all the pictures of all the former nurses there. Every day we scrubbed their faces — shined the pictures. We cleaned cupboards, we cleaned beds, that was when we were "probies", our first six months of training. You learned to clean.[27]

In the 1940s, Alice Swift also began her nursing education by, "learning to wash beds and make them. . . . That's one of the first things we learned, how to wash beds. We washed all the furniture in the room and the bedside table and the over-the-bed table."[28] She remembered:

> We had to always empty the wastebaskets. And we had a little hot water sterilizer where we had to boil our syringes and needles and sharpen them and store them in alcohol containers. We had to wash all the enema cans and rectal tubes and rubber gloves, and boil them, and we boiled all the bedpans. We had a song about bedpans. At night we'd always collect everybody's bedpans and we had to sterilize them.[29]

Despite the fact that she opted for a diploma rather than a degree course, Sally Wagner's introduction to nursing in the late 1950s was very different from that of her older colleagues. She remembered:

> We would have class all day long, and then we were expect-
> ed to work in the evening . . . another six to eight hours. . . .
> We had anatomy, microbiology, chemistry, history of nurs-
> ing, and just all the courses that I think they have now,
> except now I think when you get your bachelors degree you
> are also taking English courses and math courses. . . . This
> was five days a week, and you never had a day off during
> the week that you weren't going to class or working. A lot
> of us worked even on Saturday or Sunday for extra pay.[30]

The academic component of nursing education had grown by the
1950s, but student nurses were still expected to do a good deal of
practical work.

Although Evelyn Lantz began her nursing education in the
1930s, her introduction to nursing was different from that of the
other respondents because she was admitted to the degree program jointly offered by Brokaw Nursing School and Illinois
Wesleyan University. The program was five years long:

> You had two years at Illinois Wesleyan taking a regular
> Liberal Arts course with a . . . science major, and then you
> entered the School of Nursing (the diploma school) at
> Brokaw. Wesleyan would accept your credits from the
> diploma School of Nursing as college credits so that you got
> your degree with a major in nursing. That's what I did.

Evelyn remembers that nursing degree students were accepted
more easily by Illinois Wesleyan students than by nursing diploma
students at Brokaw:

> It was a matter of sort of like teasing — you know, "Those
> college girls, they think they're so smart" — and they would
> play tricks on us which were hurtful. I remember one of
> the little incidents. We always had dirty linen, you know,
> when you're working with patients. I was told that I had to
> wash that out by hand and carry it down to the laundry
> room and give it to the head laundry man. Of course, that
> wasn't true, but I didn't know it. It was that kind of
> thing.[31]

When Evelyn received her nursing education, degree students

were in the minority. A generation later they were in the majority, and diploma programs were either shutting down or making the transition to degree programs.

In addition to endless cleaning duties, before the introduction of inexpensive, mass-produced, disposable hospital equipment, student nurses made many of the materials used in patient care. Ruth Carpenter remembers making dressings of gauze and strips of cotton:

> We made our own cotton balls and squares, two-by-two
> squares and four-by-four squares and abdominal pads and
> then we made toothpick applicators [i.e., Q-tips]. I know I
> made enough toothpick applicators to reach from here
> [Shirley] to Bloomington twice.[32]

From the beginning of their training, nursing students trained in the first half of the twentieth century did an enormous amount of patient care. Many patients stayed in the hospital for a very long time. Ruth Carpenter recalled, "If a patient came in with pneumonia, you didn't figure he'd get out except from three weeks to four. It would take three weeks to pass the crisis. Everything took a lot longer then. They didn't have any antibiotics."[33] Medical theories and hospital customs combined to keep hospital patients in bed doing very little for themselves. Since few hospital rooms had private bathrooms, nurses passed bedpans and bathed patients in bed. They gave back rubs and sat with patients who were at risk. Jane Tinsley, who attended Brokaw's nursing school during the 1940s, described a typical day for a nursing student:

> Well, there were lots of times we did what they called split
> shifts. . . . In other words, you worked an eight hour day,
> and they usually planned your work so your class time
> wouldn't come out of your work. . . . We used to get up and
> eat, then we had chapel where you sang a couple of songs
> and had a poem read or whatever — people took turns lead-
> ing chapel. Then when we went out, we had to have a
> check of the cloth on your collar — you couldn't have your
> hair on your collar. And you went to your respective floors
> whatever they happened to be. Of course you rotated, you
> spent so many times on each floor — so much on medical,
> so much on surgical, so much in O.B.. Usually you listened
> to reports, and if you were just on a general floor, you were
> assigned so many patients to do their baths. And you did

their baths, even if they went home that afternoon, you gave them a bath. They didn't take their own bath. They washed their face, as a rule, and they "finished their bath." Other than that, you gave them their whole bath.... And then you did everything. If the individual needed an enema, they got the enema somehow worked in between all the other baths and what have you.... When I first went into training, if somebody had surgery, you made up the bed for them. They brought them down from surgery and transferred them into the bed, and then you sat with that patient in his room and took pulse and respiration until he woke up and [was] really responding and knowing what he was doing and where he was before you could leave him.[34]

Students had to learn to ignore the sights and smells of ill-health. Roberta Holman said:

I'll never forget we had this bachelor up from Lexington who had a ruptured appendix. Our rooms then were just like little bitty cubicles.... The man died, of course. We did not have penicillin.... But with dressings — the odor was so bad, we didn't have all these things to kill odor then like you do now. But I had to do it out by the door. I could not stay in the room. The odor was just horrible.[35]

Ruth Carpenter remembered that "One of the first things I had to do when I was a student was up in surgery, and they were amputating a leg, and I got to hold the leg.... They didn't have anything else to do with it. Somebody had to hold it. They didn't want to let it just fall on the floor in a floor pan."[36]

Students also had to put aside deeply inculcated feelings of maidenly modesty and shame in order to do their jobs. Roberta Holman said:

This was embarassing for 18, 19, 20-year olds. We had to prep everybody. Surgery didn't do that, and we didn't have orderlies. Now, you get in a 19, 20, 30, 35-year old man and you have to go in and do a prep for an appendectomy — it wasn't easy.[37]

In addition to such personal attention, students trained before World War II learned to administer therapies which would be regarded as very old-fashioned later in their careers. Both Ruth Carpenter, trained in the 1920s, and Evelyn Lantz, trained in the 1930s, learned to make mustard plasters. Evelyn said, "We were taught how to make a mustard plaster to the degree of redness to draw the blood to the surface as a counter-irritant. You could put it on the back if you had a headache, or on the chest. This was in our Nursing Procedures, and we were taught how to do it. I never did it for a patient."[38] Ruth had more experience with these poultices, remembering that, "Of course you had to be real careful with those. Some people, blond people, if you put too much mustard, oh, you'd get a big fat blister. Oh. You could be sicker with that than you would with what you were using the poultice for."[39]

Sally Wagner, an obstetrical nurse trained in the late 1950s, reported, "A lot of nurseries would have a bottle of whiskey so if a baby's heart rate were a little slow, or if they felt the baby needed to be stimulated a little bit, you would have an eye dropper and you would give them a couple of drops of whiskey."[40] Roberta Holman, trained during the 1940s, remembered using hot packs on the chest for pneumonia. She also administered milk molasses enemas. On one occasion, she recalled:

> Our supervisor said to one of my classmates and I, "Go up and give an enema to that [patient]. . . ." We said, "We've never been checked on enemas." She said, "It's all right 'cause you're gonna give one now. . . ." And to top it all off, it was on a fracture bed , and the man was laying here, and his bottom came through . . . . So Charlotte and I went in to give this milk molasses enema, and we did not know what to do, seeing this fat bottom down there. So, here we were, underneath the bed. We were looking at each other under there, and we'd get tickled. We were just two "probies", you know, and so we go back in this old room where we got the bedpans, and Charlotte doubles over laughing. So we go back in with a straight face and we get that tube. I make her take it, and so finally I tried, and she tried. I finally made it. I got it in, but I didn't get it in far enough. We let that old milk molasses run in the tube and out. . . . Molasses went everywhere! [41]

Students worked very long hours. Roberta Holman described the typical day of a nursing student in the late 1930s as follows:

> You didn't know what eight hours was. You went to class. . . . You put in your eight hours work . . . and then when you got further along you were on call. If they had two babies

at night, you were up with those babies and you were up on duty the next morning. They had split hours which was really bad.... You might, oh, work from 7 a.m. - 9:30, that way you could work like mad and get five baths in and then you would go to class for a couple of hours, then you would have lunch. Then you would go to class, come back and work up until 7 p.m. to do all the evening cares. I mean you would give back rubs and . . . the whole bit.[42]

Students went to school year round, and rarely had more than a half-day off at a time.

Nursing sisters experienced even greater demands on their time than lay students. Regarding her training in the 1930s, Sister Theonilla remembered:

I got up early in the morning, sisters do. We had early morning prayers together, mass together, breakfast together, and then we went on duty and nursed all day. There was no time off.
Interviewer: How long was your day?
Respondent: Until we finished in the evening. We never had any certain time we went off. You got your work done and took care of your patients. That was the main thing. . . .
Interviewer: Did you have any time off?
Respondent: Well, I didn't really. The nurses had their days off, you know. I never really did. I was always there, day and night. That was just the way it was . . . that was the sister's job. As a sister, you look at that a little different.[43]

Unlike lay students, nuns did not expect their roles to change much once they had finished their training. Change for them came in the form of increasing expertise and levels of responsibility.

To some extent, the stipends paid to student nurses helped to compensate for the long hours and unremitting work. Nursing school was as much a job as an educational program. However, beginning in the late 1920s, the amount paid to students decreased, according to Maude Essig, director of Brokaw's nursing school, "to offset the cost of instruction. During this year [1928] the case study method of learning was instituted. Graduate staff nurses were added to relieve the students of many responsibilities previously accorded to them and to provide a more stable nursing service."[44] Ruth Carpenter remembers being paid eight dollars per month during her first year, and ten dollars per month there-after.[45]

During the 1930s, both student stipends and the salaries of staff nurses were reduced because of the financial hardship caused by the Depression. However, by the time the economy improved, nurse training, in some schools at least, had begun to undergo the transition from apprenticeship to academic preparation. Evelyn Lantz says of her own class of 1938, "We were the last ones to receive a stipend. The next class that entered didn't have a stipend. I can't remember what it was, but it was just enough to pay for our books. I never had any money left over. . . . Probably around $5 - $6 per month."[46]

How did student nurses learn to do their jobs? Practical nursing was taught by staff nurses, who were universally remembered as strict and exacting in their expectations of students. Ruth Carpenter remembered Maude Essig, who was director of Brokaw Hospital's Nursing School between 1924 and 1956:

> She was very straight-laced. And she was only trying to make good nurses of us. . . . And I . . . , well, you treated her with respect. . . . She was very particular about how we kept the patients' rooms. . . . And she had certain ways that she liked the linens put in the drawers. . . . You wanted them so that the closed end was toward the drawer beginning when you opened the door. So it would be the closed end of a sheet, or a pillowcase or a towel. . . . And if you did-n't do it right you got to go do it over so you learned after awhile. . . . .She was strict. . . . Everybody liked her in a sense of the word, but she, when she said "no" and "do this," you did it that way. You didn't ask why, you just did it.[47]

Sally Wagner said of her instructors in the 1950s, "They were very professional. They were there to teach you and they expected you to learn. Some of the instructors were very strict, so they were not like a buddy-buddy-type instructor. They were all business."[48]

Student nurses practiced new skills on dummies (one at Brokaw was called "Mrs. Chase"),[49] each other, and, finally, patients. Sally Wagner remembered:

> We had clinical instructors that would sort of follow us around. . . . Each new procedure — we would be expected to demonstrate that we could do it, and they would check us

off to make sure that we knew what we were doing. We also had classroom instructions when we'd have to give each other baths, shots, wrap bandages, practice on each other, but they would also check us out on patients too. We were not expected to do it until we were okayed by the instructor. We really never had the supervision that these students have now. You know, once they checked you off on a procedure, then you were free to do it as many times as was expected.[50]

Physicians on staff did much of the clinical instruction for student nurses. Because professional nursing has traditionally been based on the authority of physicians and the deference of nurses, student nurses learned professional etiquette in addition to clinical subjects. Jane Tinsley remembered of her training in the 1940s: "And, of course, any time a doctor walked into the room you immediately stood up; they were 'God', practically."[51] Evelyn Lantz remembered that at Brokaw during the 1930s:

Dr. Markowitz was a pathologist for Brokaw Hospital, and he had his own independent office in pathology. He was the best teacher. . . . Then we had Dr. Brian and Dr. Jenkins to teach us surgical conditions. Dr. Doud taught us obstetrics. . . . Oh, I forgot Ed Stevenson, he taught us medical too. . . . He was a very good teacher. He liked to tell us how much he knew too, but he was also a very good teacher. He had a very short temper. When you made rounds with him, you had better know exactly what you are doing. . . . All the doctors that we had in my experience at Brokaw in the School of Nursing had high regard for the students, and when we graduated every doctor gave us a gift.[52]

Sally Wagner was also taught by hospital staff physicians during her training at Grant Hospital School in Chicago during the late 1950s:

They were very good teachers and they expected you to listen. When the doctor talked everybody just was quiet and he would make rounds. The interns and residents would go and the [nursing] students would go and he would teach at the bedside. He would come to the patient and he would tell us what the problems were in front of the patient and he would say what he was going to do, and . . . then he would ask questions to the interns and residents, but the nurses were never asked questions. We were just there to learn.[53]

As time went on, students took an increasing amount of academic course work with university faculty members, although Alice Swift remembered that, "Our books were tiny compared to what the students have now. They weren't hard at all. . . . The books were so simple and easy compared to college."[54]

In addition, students' educations were enhanced by clinical rotations at hospitals with which their nursing schools had developed affiliations. Ruth Carpenter studied pediatrics at a hospital in Indianapolis. Evelyn Lantz recalled:

> We affiliated with Milwaukee Children's Hospital and the nurses taught us pediatrics. We did not have doctors teaching us. The courses were all taught by nurses. Then we affiliated with Peoria State Hospital, which is in Bartonville, for our psychiatric work. We had physicians teach us there and the Nursing Arts Instructor taught us how to care for what we had to do . . . .[55]

Generally speaking, nurses remembered these experiences as highlights of their training. For many, it was the first time they had been far from home; thus, the experience was liberating. It could also be frightening. One respondent remembered of her rotation at Bartonville:

> I was scared to death when I first went over there. I almost got kicked out of training, too, over there. . . . I was pretty much a home-body. To be gone and not be able to see my folks and stay all night with them for six months was unheard-of, you know. So Abby and I decided we were going to go home. . . . We were dressed and in bed, and after this mean old woman checked us at night, we went out a window. . . . We thumbed a ride, got into the car with some drunks, we were scared to death, and there was a tavern down the way, so we told them we wanted a drink . . . would they buy us a drink. So they stopped at this tavern, and we had to go to the restroom. We walked right out of that building, went out, thumbed a ride and got a ride home. . . . The next day at class the teacher said, "I understand there were two girls who hitchiked to Bloomington,

and I have no idea who it was." Of course they didn't! There was only two there from Bloomington. "And unless they report to us immediately, they will be expelled from school." We about knocked those people over getting up there. We were — what is it you call it? — we couldn't leave, we couldn't go anywhere the rest of the time we were there. Anyway, it's a part of growing up.[56]

Nursing school rules were strict, designed to protect both the young women who attended them and their reputations. Ruth Carpenter recalled that Brokaw's regulations were a bit more relaxed than Mennonite's in the 1920s. However, they were demanding by today's standards:

Well, you didn't get married. That was the head of the list. You didn't get married because if you did, you went out on your toot. And you had to be in at 10:00. And, if you were on call, you couldn't leave the campus. Your boyfriend could come to see you if he wanted to, but you couldn't leave the campus. And you had to go to Chapel and . . . our uniforms had to be halfway respectable looking. . . . We didn't wear jewelry. No earrings. None of that sort of thing. No jewelry in uniform. And we didn't smoke in uniform. . . . And you didn't wear your cap off campus.[57]

Even in the 1950s, student nurses' behavior was closely controlled.[58]

Student nurses lived in the hospital, in purpose-designed residence halls, or in private homes supervised by housemothers. In early years, before hospital expansion programs increased available space, student accommodations were a low priority. Jennie Miller, who graduated from Brokaw Hospital's School of Nursing in 1906, remembered, "When the nurses lived on the top floor of the old Brokaw building, there was such a dire need for patient beds that the nurses moved into tents on the hospital lawn. We undressed in the hospital and scooted out to the tents in our night clothes."[59] Not until May Mecherle Hall was constructed in 1941 did Brokaw's student nurses have purpose-built accommodations. Mennonite's student nurses were housed in private homes until 1946, when the Troyer Memorial Nurses' Home opened its doors.

Despite hard work, strict discipline, and rather spartan living conditions, nurses remembered their training with nostalgia.

Many made firm friendships; all remembered good times. Ruth Carpenter said:

> We had a lot of fun. My roommate, she was as crazy as I was so we got along real well together. She had an old ukelele and of a night we'd come off duty, maybe in the summertime, and we lived on the Southwest corner..., and we had a fire escape outside of our room. So we decided we'd have a concert. So she got her ukelele out and I and all the rest of us had combs with tissue or toilet paper on them and we had a concert out on the little patio there, the fire escape.... And there was a nurse, and she was a World War I nurse, and she was very sedate; straight-laced as all get out.... And, oh, she raised Cain, but the patients just loved it.[60]

Graduate Nurses

Nurse training ended with graduation and licensing. This involved taking a state board examination. Nurses moving to Illinois from other states had to become licensed in Illinois before obtaining employment. Sister Theonilla was first licensed in Iowa. She remembered:

> I got licensed in three states: Iowa, Illinois and Michigan....
> *Interviewer*: So when you moved you had to take a licensing exam?
> *Respondent*: Yeah. From Springfield.... You had to fill out some papers and then sign your name, and with a doctor's signature. Then I got my license.[61]

Licenses were renewed annually. Local nursing organizations provided an opportunity for graduate nurses to stay in contact with each other and upgrade their skills.

Before the late 1940s, most graduate nurses went into private duty nursing. In the early years of the century, this work was comparatively well-paid. In 1920, Brokaw Hospital's "Registry Rules" listed the following fees for services:

> $42.00 per week for general nursing
> $7.00 per day for quarantine cases, mental, nervous, genito-urinary and last stages of carcinoma and tuberculosis

$7.00 per day for pneumonia and typhoid through critical period, and $6.00 per day through convalescence
$7.00 per day for obstetrics
$10.00 per call for assisting with delivery
$42.00 per week from date of engagement to confinement
$5.00 to $10.00 for assisting with operations in the home
This fee in addition to charge if nurse remains on case
$10.00 per week or $2.00 per day for each additional patient
When two nurses are employed, each shall charge the regular fee.
Nurses are entitled to six hours rest at night and three or four hours off for recreation each day.
Traveling expenses including taxicab when needed at night to be paid by employer.

Graduate nurses who were members of their nursing school alumnae organizations and the Sixth District Illinois Nurses' Association were eligible for the hospital's registry. In addition, nurses accepted private duty jobs at the invitation of physicians.

During the Depression years of the 1930s, private duty work became less readily available and fees declined. Ruth Carpenter explained, "Nurses were a dime a dozen. You couldn't hardly find a job." When she graduated in 1931, Ruth took a room in a house where she could work for her board and room when she was not nursing. She put her name on the private duty register at Brokaw Hospital, "and maybe you'd get a case for three days, and then when you got off that case you'd go right down to the bottom of the register."[62] When she did get work, Ruth was unhappy about the working conditions, calling private duty "a slave driver's trade. You'd work 20 hours for six dollars. Now, that's not much money. . . . And in 1931 and '32 people did not have private duty nurses unless they were just desperately ill. And you'd watch them, and we worked 20-hour shifts."[63]

Shortly after finishing her training, Ruth was asked to take an erysipelas case by Dr. Minnick of Danvers, who picked her up with his horse and buggy to drive her to the patient's home:

Well, this man was shaving one Sunday morning and there was a little pimple . . . right close to his nose. And by the end of the day, it began to get . . . worse. So the family was, they were not rich but they were affluent enough they could afford to . . . have somebody to come to the house.

And he [Dr. Minnick] came in to get me and he said, "What were you trained to use for erysipelas?" And I said, "Well, the only thing I ever knew was hot Epsom salt packs." So ... it took us three weeks to get this man well, but we got him well. ... And of course it's an awful disease. It used to many times be fatal.[64]

Ruth also assisted with home deliveries during the 1930s, learning to bake linens in the oven to sterilize them and to use a portable delivery table. On one occasion:

This young man came to me in the middle of the night and he said, "Mrs. Carpenter, my momma is in confinement. Will you come and help her?" The aunt was going to do it, and they got pretty far along and discovered the cord was around the neck about two times, so I went out and helped.[65]

Working conditions for both hospital staff and private duty nurses eased in 1937 when the Women's Eight Hour Law was implemented. Ruth Carpenter commented that, "The doctors were sure that the patients would all die. They didn't think anybody could live with two nurses."[66] Nonetheless, physicians, nurses and patients accommodated to the new regulations.

Conditions were somewhat better when Roberta Holman did private duty nursing after she graduated in the 1940s:

I took special Mrs. W.H. Roland in her home out at Country Club Place. That was in 1946-47. ... Dr. Ed Stevenson called me and asked me if I would go take care of her. ... And I took care of her for several months. I was pregnant. . . at that time, and it was really nice working in a home like that. ... So that was a good experience . . . . [But] finally I think I was getting on her nerves and she was definitely getting on my nerves. She had cancer, you know, and was very ill. And so I called Dr. Ed Stevenson and I said, "You know, I think she's getting tired of me and I'm getting tired, period." And I said I would really like to be relieved.[67]

At this time, nursing jobs were easy to find; indeed, Roberta selected private duty to suit her own convenience.

In the early twentieth century, hospital staff positions were

140

available only to nursing's elite — unmarried women who had been trained in a small number of highly regarded nursing schools. A letter sent to an applicant for the position of surgical nurse at Brokaw Hospital in 1907 indicates contemporary working conditions and personnel structure:

My dear Miss Hartley,

I send you under separate cover a circular of our Hospital. We can accommodate nearly fifty [patients], at present we have twenty-four. Some days we have two and three operations, then again for several days we may have none.

My surgical nurse assists me with the housekeeping. We have two floor maids, cook, waitress and laundress. We send our flat work to the steam laundry.

The Surgical Nurse has a pupil assistant who assists her for a term of two months in the operating room. At the present time we have a very capable pupil nurse assisting, and I will keep her on for two weeks in October to assist the newcomer. At present, my surgical nurse is one of our own graduates and has completed a year's services. She is quite anxious to take up private nursing, hence her resignation.

Our work is general, and our nursing corps consists of myself; my first assistant who has charge of the nursing and is a graduate of the Henrietta Hospital of East St. Louis, Miss Justis, also took post-graduate work at the Presbyterian Hospital of Chicago, and is a very agreeable, capable woman. I have a graduate night head nurse, who has a pupil with her on each floor. I hardly think you could be more agreeably located in any small place. . . .

The salary is $40.00 per month with expenses . . . . I would like to have someone come by the first of October. We might say for three months, then I would like to have you stay the year through if we are mutually suited. It might interest you to know that two graduate nurses from your school are located here. Miss Ellen Charles and Miss Emma Bluhm.[68]

Staff nurses lived in the hospital. They tended to leave their positions, either for the relative freedom of private duty nursing or to marry.

Like private duty nurses, staff nurses suffered during the

Depression. When Ruth Carpenter found private duty nursing an unreliable source of income, she worked for a time as a staff nurse at Brokaw. She reported:

> Times were rough. We had about five general duty nurses then. And she [Miss Essig] brought us all in for a meeting and she said, "Now, I'm either going to have to lay some of you off or everybody take a cut." So we decided we had board, room and laundry. Now, you can't hardly beat that. . . . [We] took the cut. I made fifty-five dollars a month.[69]

However, after the beginning of World War II, the demand for all types of medical professionals mushroomed.

The federal government responded to the need for military nurses by sponsoring the Nurses' Cadet program. In 1944, a Nurses' Cadet Corps was set up at Mennonite Hospital. Students involved in this program had their expenses paid and received stipends in return for the commitment that they would remain active nurses for the duration of the war.[70] After the war ended in 1945, the need for nurses continued.

In 1946, with veterans returning from military service; wives quitting work to look after families; and the Baby Boom getting underway, McLean County discovered that it had a shortage of nurses. Hospital utilization was increasing, while enrollment in nurse training programs was declining. A newspaper report indicated:

> 1) Each of the three hospitals needs to double its present nursing staff: 2) The nurse per patient ratio is approximately 1 to 7 in Bloomington-Normal, whereas the normal ratio is 1 to 3: and 3) fewer students are entering nurses training now.[71]

The Nurses Recruitment Committee set up by Brokaw, Mennonite and St. Joseph's hospitals established the goal of attracting 125 nursing students to local training programs in the autumn of 1946. In addition, local hospitals began hiring graduate nurses under more favorable conditions than those prevailing earlier in the century. Wages increased and the requirement that staff nurses be unmarried and live in hospitals was quietly dropped. Like school teaching, nursing became a realistic life-long career opportunity.

The Post-War Years

In the second half of the twentieth century, most professional nursing has been done in institutional settings. Hospitals became the major employers, with doctor's offices, factories, schools and public health departments also contributing to a growing demand for nurses. Like professional medicine, nursing became increasingly specialized and dependent upon an expanding range of technologies and equipment. According to one historian,

> The increasingly technical and machine-aided nature of hospital-based health care has . . . affected nursing's situation. Nurses are now responsible for an array of new technologies and procedures from cardiac-monitoring devices to respiratory therapies. . . . Nursing, after all, is what is intensive about intensive-care units.[72]

These changes occurring on a national level also affected nursing in McLean County. Jane Tinsley, who went into public health nursing, commented:

> We got more specialized, not only in the hospital setting, but also in public health and some of the other agencies, in school nursing and what have you. All of a sudden they have blood pressure monitoring and . . . heart monitoring where you are reading all these machines. Well, that was just unheard of . . . . If you had heard about this when I was in training here, it would have been like Buck Rogers in the 20th Century. Unbelievable.[73]

According to Sister Theonilla,

> Nursing has changed in a lot of ways. It's more complicated.
> *Interviewer*: In what respect is it more complicated?
> *Respondent*: Well, all the equipment that you have nowadays, and the medications are much more involved. . . . And the IVs — all that. It's not what it used to be. And the treatment of the patients too is different.[74]

Nurses agree that these changes have both positive and

negative aspects. According to Roberta Holman,

> Well, I think they [nurses] know so much more, or there's so
> much more for them to do. I mean, it's just progress. All of
> the machines and all of the fantastic things they can do
> now for people. But I think the nurses will tell you that we
> don't get the good bedside nursing. A nurse really doesn't
> give bedside nursing any more. And patients miss the bed-
> side — they need that.[75]

Respondents agreed that while more nurses have degrees
and advanced skills, they spend less time giving hands-on patient
care. Sister Theonilla criticized this trend in nursing:

> I don't think it takes a master's and doctorate degree to
> take care of a patient. What they need is a lot of good care
> and tender loving care. They don't need initials. As long as
> you know what you are doing and are responsible for what
> you're doing: that's the main thing, I think.[76]

Nurses' work changed in other ways. As the salaries and
status of nurses increased, hospitals added to their housekeeping
staffs and stopped expecting nurses to scrub buildings, clean
instruments, do laundry and make beds. In addition, with the
development of disposable equipment, nurses no longer had to
make their own or clean it for further use. Sister Theonilla
remembered that early in her career:

> We made all those things. . . . You took cotton and rolled it
> up into balls. . . . You made all your bandages. You just
> bought a ball of cotton and a ball of gauze.
> *Interviewer*: Did all the nurses do this?
> *Respondent*: Yeah. All together. There was a big supply on
> the [surgical] unit, you know. We didn't have a supply
> downstairs to go and get, we had to make them. . ..I think
> that is an . . . expensive change. . . . Things come now
> already sterilized in a package and if you don't use the
> whole package, well you can't use it any more. . . . We
> washed our instruments, too, that weren't used. . ... There
> was nothing disposable. . . . Like IV tubings, and all
> that. . . . That was a job to clean.[77]

144

Nurses also became responsible for an increasing amount of paperwork. Sister Theonilla said, "I think there is too much paperwork. Paperwork, well some of it is necessary; you have to keep accurate records. Sometimes you need to look back at that if a patient is having problems. But then, it's overdone I think."[78]

In the years after World War II, with enhancement of the academic component in nursing education and development of the Women's Movement, relationships between nurses and physicians also changed. Evelyn Lantz, born in the 1930s, had pleasant memories of the physicians who taught student nurses at Brokaw:

> Many of those men felt they had a father/daughter relationship, and they felt that they sort of needed to take care of us. . . . It was a very, I don't want to use the word "patronizing", but it was a family kind of thing.[79]

Alice Swift's memories of the relationships between doctors and nurses in the early years of her career were less pleasant:

> It was not as comfortable to be in nursing in large hospitals unless nurses knew how to assert themselves well. . . .
> Doctors were very abusive. They continued to be for a long time, as far as I was concerned. They liked to blame things on nurses. . . .
> *Interviewer*: How have nurse/physician relationships changed over the years?
> *Respondent*: It depends on where you're located as far as I can see. And on your position. When you go over to [nearby community], the interaction there is much more collegial that in was here in this community. . . . Here, nurses were not treated as well as they were over there. Primary nursing put the nurse in a very different posture. It took an awful lot of strength in a nurse to know how to deal with some of the treatment doctors handed out.[80]

Jane Tinsley said about her own early nursing experience:

> Fewer doctors thanked you and made you feel like you were appreciated. Lots of times you felt like you were the invisible person there doing the job. He wanted it, and it was expected, and it should be ready. You anticipated. Some of them did appreciate what the nurse did. Many of them gave the feeling that the service was their due — they had studied and put in all the time and "I'm saving this individual's life."[81]

Roberta Holman reflected on the change in the relationship between nurses and doctors during her career:

> It was different then because, you know, they [nurses] were kind of the underdog as far as doctors were concerned. I mean, when a doctor walked in a room you jumped up because if you didn't you would be reprimanded. We looked up to the doctors like they were gods. Not anymore. Nurses got smart. You know they [doctors] are human beings just like everybody else.[82]

Sally Wagner, a generation younger, made a similar comment. Early in her career:

> Even if you were busy doing something like charting . . . you always stood up, and you never entered the room before them. You always let the doctors go into the room before you did. . . . I think now . . . most doctors stand back and let the nurses go into the room before they enter, so I think . . . it's a little more of an equal respect now than just one way. . . . I think it's different today. I think the doctors treat the nurses much better. I think they are on a social level too. They include us in some of their social activities. We know their families, they know our families. . . .[83]

Another significant change in nursing after about 1960 was the increasing diversity of both nursing student bodies and professional nursing. Before this time, in McLean County, nursing schools were attended exclusively by young white women, most of whom came from rural or small town backgrounds. Neither non-whites nor men were accepted. When Betty Ebo, an African American resident of Bloomington, applied to St. Joseph's Nursing School in 1944, despite the national shortage of nurses she was refused admission because, "We've never taken a colored student."[84] She obtained her training from the all-black nursing school run by St. Mary's Infirmary in St. Louis, later becoming a Dominican nun. St. Joseph's began training African American nursing students in the 1950s; Mennonite awarded its diploma to the first African American in 1978. The first male nursing student, Kenneth Unzicker, graduated from the Mennonite Hospital

School of Nursing in 1963. In the last quarter of the twentieth century, nursing, like professional medicine, has benefited from increasing racial and gender tolerance and from affirmative action legislation.

Conclusions

More than any other occupation, except perhaps military service, nursing is inextricably linked to prevailing ideas about gender roles. Nurses must still deal with the potential contradiction between being good women and successful professionals. Despite many changes, nursing is still a dominantly female profession and continues to be associated with women's social position and their presumed "natural" talent for care-giving. Nurses face the ongoing challenges of balancing professional aspirations with traditional deference to physicians, on the one hand, and the needs of patients, on the other. The history of nursing is the history of the ways those challenges have been met — with the formation of professional organizations to advocate the interests of nurses; development of rigorous training programs to improve their skills and earning power; and individual hard work earning the respect of physicians and patients.

The history of nursing in McLean County represents national developments in microcosm. From their roots in hospital-based diploma schools established to provide hospitals with an inexpensive labor force drawn from the local area, the County's nursing degree programs have become both academically rigorous and nationally competitive, attracting students from other states and foreign countries. In contrast to the earlier local pattern of graduate nurses either doing private duty nursing or stopping paid work when they married, nursing has truly become a life-long career option offering a range of professional opportunities. Finally, the status of nurses in the county has altered from that of a skilled and respectable servant to that of an independent expert with exclusive competencies.

Nonetheless, some things have not changed. In McLean County as elsewhere, nurses are still expected to put the needs of their patients before their own. They are expected to deal with human misery with good cheer and common sense. They are required to suspend their own judgement in favor of physicians' decisions. They remain, thus, appropriate symbols of the character of a good woman.

To Do No Harm: Healing in the Twentieth Century

It is not only for the sick man, it is for the sick man's friends that the Doctor comes. His presence is often as good for them as for the patient, and they long for him yet more eagerly. How we have all watched after him! What an emotion the thrill of his carriage-wheels in the street, and at length at the door, has made us feel! How we hang upon his words, and what a comfort we get from a smile or two, if he can vouchsafe that sunshine to lighten our darkness! . . . Over the patient in fever, the wife expectant, the children unconscious, the doctor stands as if he were Fate, the dispenser of life and death.

William Makepeace Thackeray, <u>History of Pendennis</u>, vol. 2 (1850)

I swear by Apollo the physician, and by Asklepios, Hygeia and Panacea, and all the gods and goddesses, and call them to witness that . . . I will prescribe treatment to the best of my ability and judgment for the good of the sick, and never for a harmful or illicit purpose. I will give no poisonous drug, even if asked to, nor make any such suggestion. . . . I will both live and work in purity and godliness. . . .
Anything I see or hear about people, whether in the course of my practice or outside it, that should not be made public, I will keep to myself and treat as an inviolable secret. . . .

From *The Hippocratic Oath* (c. 400 BC)

The professional practice of medicine is built on a marriage between the doctor's skill and the patient's trust. The physician's skill is a product of training, experience, and knowledge of the patient's circumstances. The patient's trust is born of desperation and perception of the doctor's authority. Although physicians have exercised a healing role in Western societies since ancient times, they did not have a monopoly over medical information and health care delivery until relatively recently. Popular belief in the knowledge and expertise of physicians was given an enormous boost by late nineteenth- and twentieth-century fascination with science. As front-line agents of scientific progress, doctors' power over birth, disease and death was believed to be far greater that it actually was at the turn of the century.

In 1900, surgical therapies were more effective than they had been even twenty years earlier. "Listerian" surgical procedures had made operations safer; thus, more ambitious procedures were performed. Appendectomy, pioneered in the 1880s, had become routine, as had tonsillectomy, which was increasingly done in an effort to prevent the devastating infections which threatened young life before the advent of antibiotics. Dr. William Halsted, chief surgeon at Johns Hopkins University, wrote in 1910:

> Consider the every-day, urgent problems which have been confronting the surgeon — problems involving the life of the patient — and which each actively engaged surgeon has in great part had to solve or try to solve for himself. The recognition and treatment of appendicitis, of affections of the bile passages, of the pancreas, of the kidneys. The devising of the various forms of intestinal suture, the cure of hernia, of cancer, of exophthalmic goiter. The treatment of the enlarged prostate gland, recognition and treatment of diverticula of the bladder and oesophagus, of ulcer and cancer of the stomach. The management of hemorrhage, the surgery of the arteries and veins, and in general the entire surgery of the abdominal, thoracic and cranial cavities, I might almost say of the whole body. Twenty years ago we did not know how to close an abdominal wound, nor how to make one. And as to technique, surgeons throughout the world operated, little more than ten years ago, not only without gloves or other protection, but in their everyday clothes, covered usually by a rubber apron taken from a hook and used day after day and week after week without sterilization.[1]

Nonetheless, even taking account of such advances, surgery would become a much more powerful therapeutic instrument in the twentieth century, benefiting enormously from innovations in technology, biochemistry and pharmacology.

Medical therapies lagged behind surgery. Although the germ theory was well established by the end of the nineteenth century, with the exception of a few antitoxins no truly powerful agents had yet been developed to combat the infections that still caused great mortality. Thus, prevention was far more powerful than medicine, and doctors tended to become involved only after patients had become seriously ill. Old humoral treatments, mainly intended to produce evacuation, continued to be used. Physicians were called upon for advice and moral support. However, they, like worried family members, were often powerless against disease. Those rejecting old-fashioned remedies and treatment regimes were often forced into a passive role, watching and waiting as an illness ran its course.

In 1900, most physicians were prepared for medical practice by brief academic training programs enhanced by extensive clinical practice, first supervised by an experienced practitioner, then carried on independently. The doctor's reputation was based upon his (or, in some cases, her) relationships with patients and their families. It was fostered by an appropriate demeanor and participation in community activities. A physician's reputation was not necessarily dependent on success, since most illnesses were reckoned to be beyond the power of man to cure. Rather, doctors were consulted because their medical knowledge and expertise were believed to be superior to the healing abilities of lay people. They were also often the last resort of people who had first tried other ways of dealing with illness.

During the last quarter of the nineteenth century, most states began to regulate the practice of medicine. Faced with the reality of widely varying quality in the hodgepodge of medical schools then operating in the state, Illinois' Medical Practice Act of 1877 resolved:

> That on and after July 1, 1878, the Board will not consider any medical college in good standing which holds two graduating courses in one year. Also, that . . . the Board will not recognize the diplomas of any medical school which does not require of its candidates for graduation the actual attendance upon at least two full courses of lectures at an interval of six months or more.[2]

Older practitioners or those with diplomas from unrecognized schools could obtain licenses to practice by taking an examination. Revised several times before licensing of physicians was transferred from the State Board of Health to the Department of Registration and Education in 1917, legislation regulating the practice of medicine took into account changing standards regarding medical education and changing expectations of medical care on the part of the general public. Minimum educational prerequisites for medical study were identified and extended; examinations continued to be administered to practitioners who were not graduates of schools which conformed to increasingly stringent state curriculum requirements.[3]

In the course of the twentieth century, both the power of professional medicine and patients' expectations of health care mushroomed. As therapeutics caught up with scientific discoveries, medical and surgical treatments became increasingly successful. As medical knowledge grew, specialists carved out increasingly exclusive spheres of operation. The partnership between doctors and hospitals, tentative in the early years of the century, dominated professional health care after about 1950. Twentieth-century American medical care has, thus, been characterized by a focus on acute care delivered in institutional environments where the tools of modern medicine and surgery are most effective. The transformation of medical education is of central significance in these changes, both reflecting and stimulating them.

Reform of Medical Education

The twentieth century witnessed rapid and dramatic changes in the composition and structure of the medical profession. Under pressure from professional organizations, elite physicians, and university faculties, medical education was increasingly standardized, as were criteria for licenses to practice. In contrast to the unregulated medical marketplace of nineteenth century America, in the twentieth century training programs became increasingly rigorous and entry to the profession was strictly controlled.

There was a good deal of room for improvement. Nineteenth-century American medical schools were generally regarded as vastly inferior to their European counterparts. Indeed, until the mid-twentieth century, physicians who were serious about their own preparation for practice routinely enhanced their medical educations by traveling to European centers of expertise. In the early 1870s, Charles Eliot, President of Harvard, wrote, "The ignorance and general incompetency of the average graduate of American Medical Schools, at the time when he receives the degree which turns him loose upon the community, is something horrible to contemplate. . . . The whole system of medical education in this country needs thorough reformation."[4] Eliot, who was a trained chemist, reorganized medical education at

Harvard by extending the traditional two-year program to three, requiring specific educational prerequisites for entrance, enhancing didactic lectures with laboratory training, and paying salaries to professors rather than allowing them to collect fees directly from students.[5]

Other elite institutions followed Harvard's lead during the 1880s, but the medical school established at Johns Hopkins University in 1893 set a new, still higher standard. According to one expert, "From the outset, Johns Hopkins embodied a conception of medical education as a field of graduate study, rooted in basic science and hospital medicine, that was eventually to govern all institutions in the country."[6] Entering students were required to have college degrees; graduates completed a four-year program of medical study.

Initially, the reforms initiated at universities such as Harvard, Johns Hopkins, and University of Pennsylvania served only to widen the gap between well and poorly trained physicians. Despite new state licensing laws, passed during the 1870s and 1880s, the many commercial medical schools continued to turn out large numbers of indifferently prepared (or completely unprepared) graduates who hung out their shingles and learned by doing.[7] Some of these schools simply sold diplomas. In 1910, Rush Medical College received the following letter from a self-educated doctor who was under the impression that the college operated a mail order business:

> Please accept of My hand writting though I hav'nt been in touch with you as to write you before.
> But at this time I write you for a Diploma of being a family Doctor. I have purchase a family Medical Book From Sears Roebuck and I have Studied it for two (2) years and I have been Examined by Doctor — and I Desires to Give Rush Medical College Honor for what I know, and that is why I asked for a Diploma from that College. I have been Teaching for twelve (12) years and I believe I am Prepaired to do the work. I will give you One Dollar and a half ($1.50) for the Diploma if you will Except of My request Please let Me hear from you by return Mail.[8]

At the turn of the century, there were grounds for concern on the part of commercial medical schools that the decision to raise admission standards, improve the curriculum and lengthen the period of study might drive prospective students away and into the waiting arms of less demanding schools. However, the survival of these schools was doomed by the American Medical Association's determination to raise the standards of medical education and practice. In 1904 the AMA established a Council on Medical Education which:

> formulated a minimum standard for physicians calling for four years of high school, an equal period of medical training, and passage of a licensing test; its "ideal" standard stipulated five years of medical school (including one year of basic sciences, later pushed into the "premedical" curriculum in college) and a sixth of hospital internship.[9]

The Council also inspected and graded the 160 American medical schools then in existence, categorizing just over half of them as Class A (fully approved), 29 percent as Class B (imperfect), and one-fifth as Class C (unsalvageable).[10]

Under pressure from the AMA, state licensing authorities, and university-based educational reformers, between 1906 and 1910 almost one-fifth of the weaker American medical schools closed their doors. These schools, which were generally private and without access to university or hospital facilities, could not offer the laboratory training or range of clinical experience provided by university-based medical programs. Furthermore, as the medical academic year lengthened from four to eight or nine months, and the period of training extended from two to four or more years past high school, costs increased. Schools were compelled to charge higher tuition; students and faculty members lost the earnings opportunities shorter training had provided. As a result, medical students were drawn from increasingly prosperous families with increasingly sophisticated expectations regarding medical school programs. As medical education began to require an ever greater time and financial commitment, numbers of applicants for medical schools dropped, but their educational qualifications and social status increased. An emerging consensus about the necessary characteristics of high quality preparation for medical practice, including extensive university education, laboratory-based training in the basic sciences, and hospital-based clinical experience, paved the way for the reception of the Flexner Report in 1910.

Abraham Flexner was a young educator with a bachelor's degree from Johns Hopkins University. He was commissioned by the Carnegie Foundation for the Advancement of Teaching to con-

154

duct an investigation of American medical schools and make recommendations for their reform. His report indicated that, while excellent medical education was available in the United States, most of the nation's medical schools were inadequate. He identified a yawning gap between progress in medical science and stagnation in medical education, recommending a closer association between scientific research and medical training. Flexner also recommended closure of most of the schools he visited (100 of 131), and reform of the remaining institutions on the Johns Hopkins model.[11]

Reform never went as far as Flexner or the AMA wished. Flexner's recommendations would have left a significant number of states without medical schools — an unacceptable situation.[12] However, dramatic change did come. The approximately 70 surviving medical schools embraced a model of medical education more closely associated with research than practice. This transformation was supported by major foundations which poured money into medical schools with the intention of making them into medical research centers.[13]

The reform of medical education created tension between academic physicians, who believed that scientific training was the most important component of medical education, and clinicians who felt that the medicine of university laboratories and teaching hospitals was unacceptably remote from the conditions of practice most medical graduates would face. Some advocated a two-tiered system where medical researchers would be trained at a small number of elite institutions, while the bulk of practitioners would receive more practical, clinically based educations.

Despite such concerns, American medical education became standardized, with students at all schools pursuing essentially identical curricula. As a result, those completing increasingly lengthy and rigorous medical training were imbued with a homogenous *esprit de corps* and world view. Upon graduation, they also immediately assumed a high degree of authority with patients and qualified for social status and financial rewards which increased dramatically after World War II.

Reform of medical education had a significant impact on the socioeconomic composition of professional medicine. In the highly competitive late nineteenth-century marketplace of medical education, where instruction was cheap and admission requirements lax, diversity had increased. Immigrants, African Americans and women had joined the ranks of physicians in increasing numbers. In the second half of the nineteenth century, seventeen medical colleges for women and seven for blacks were established in the United States. Many evening schools opened to offer medical training to people who needed to work during the day. However, in the early twentieth century, this trend was reversed. By 1910, only three women's medical colleges and two medical schools for African Americans remained open.[14] Unable to meet requirements for laboratory and clinical study, evening schools closed their doors. After 1910, medical schools became increasingly exclusive, limiting admission of blacks, women, and other socially undesirable groups; thus, the social composition and outlook of the medical profession became increasingly uniform. Not until after World War II would the GI Bill and the Civil Rights and Women's movements stimulate greater diversity among medical students and physicians.

Preparation for Medical Practice in McLean County

In McLean County, as in other parts of the United States, the impact of national changes came slowly and almost imperceptibly. Leaders of professional medicine during the first half of the twentieth century were mature adults who had been educated long before reform began. For example, Dr. Ernest Mammen, president of the McLean County Medical Society in 1909 and 1910, was born in 1855 and graduated from Rush Medical College in 1884. At this time, Rush's three-year curriculum depended almost entirely upon lectures. There was no laboratory-based instruction until the 1890s, and the school suffered from chronic difficulties in obtaining cadavers for dissection. While Rush examined prospective students in elementary physical science and arithmetic, there were no standard requirements for admission. An age contemporary of Dr. Mammen's, Dr. James B. Herrick, "recalled that in his class of 1888 only seven of 135 men entering the school boasted a college diploma of any description."[15] Following the conventional pattern for the well trained physician of his day, nine years after beginning practice in Bloomington, Dr. Mammen augmented his training by spending a year studying with surgical specialists in Berlin.[16]

Dr. William M. Young, president of the McLean County Medical Society in 1920, also belonged to an older medical generation. Born in 1867, he received his medical diploma in 1897 from the Eclectic Medical Institute, which closed shortly thereafter. He practiced as a general practitioner and anesthetist until his death in 1939.[17]

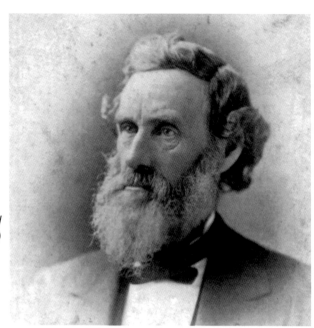

Dr. Cyrenius Wakefield
(1815 - 1885)

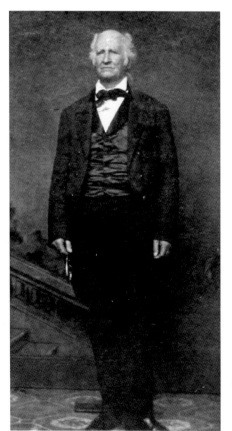

Dr. E.. G. Covington
(1872 - 1929)

Dr. John F. Henry
(1793 - 1873)

Sources for illustrations: McLean County Historical Society, Bloomington, Illinois.

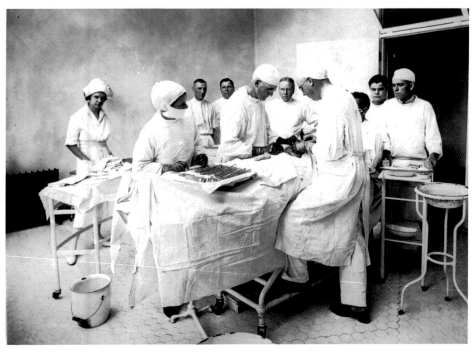

Brokaw Hospital, Surgery ca. 1922

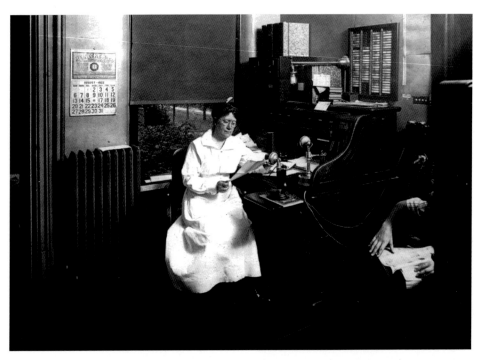

Hospital Administration In The Early Twentieth Century

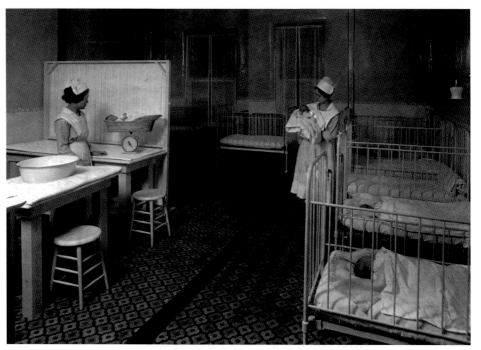

Brokaw Hospital, Maternity Ward ca. 1922

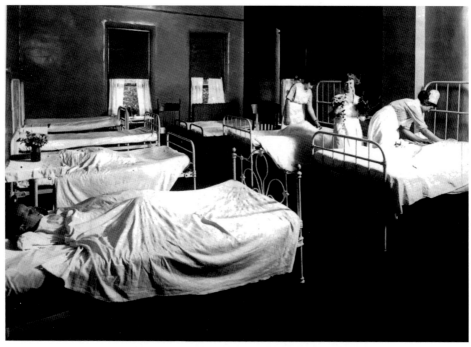

Brokaw Hospital, Children's Ward ca. 1922

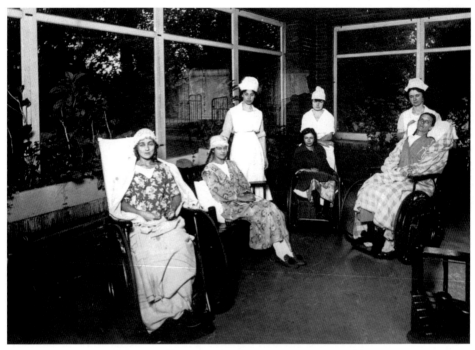

Group of Patients, Brokaw Hospital ca. 1922

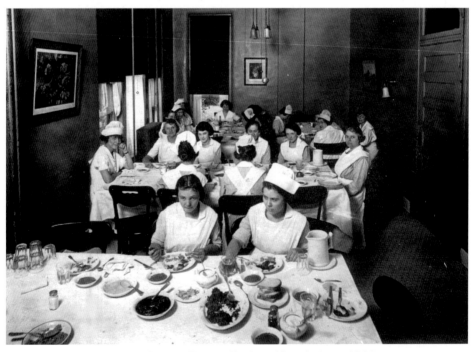

Nurses' Dining Room, Brokaw Hospital ca. 1922

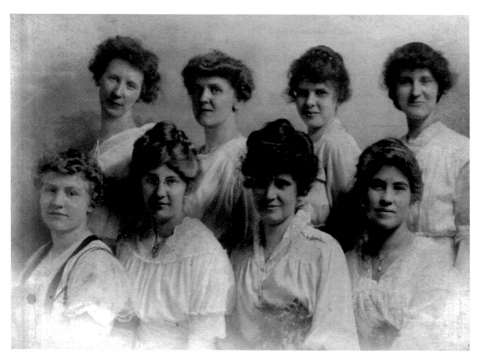

Brokaw Hospital Nursing Class ca. 1910

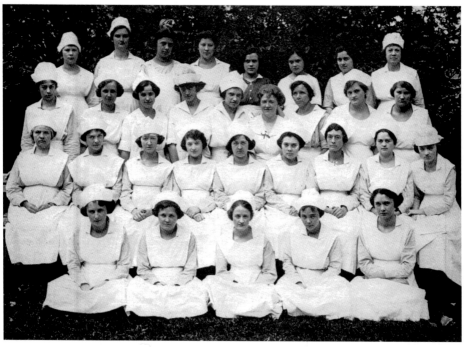

Brokaw Hospital Nursing School, Class of 1915

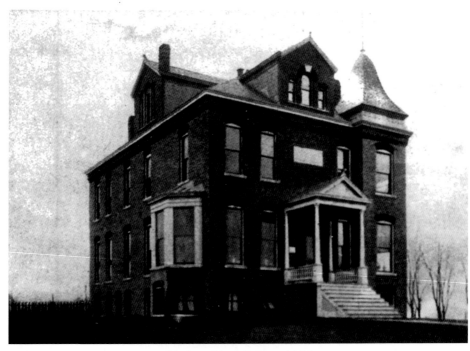

Brokaw Hospital ca. 1900

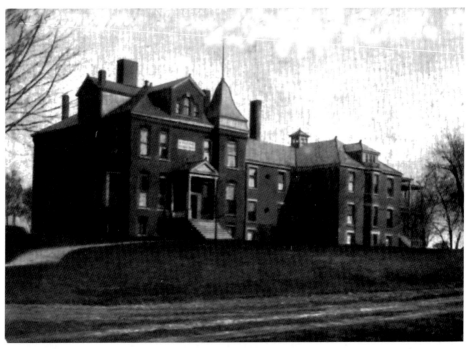

Brokaw Hospital, 1907

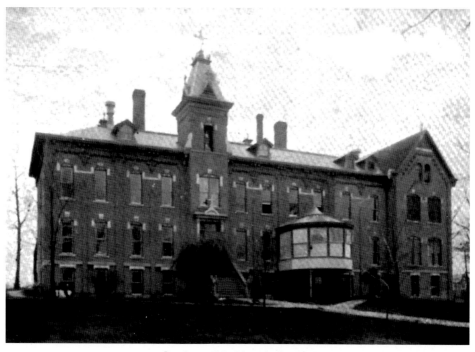

St. Joseph's Hospital, 1906

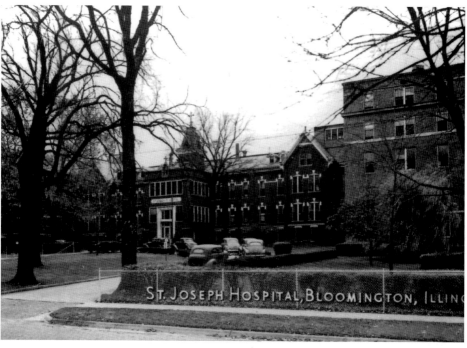

St. Joseph's Hospital ca. 1940

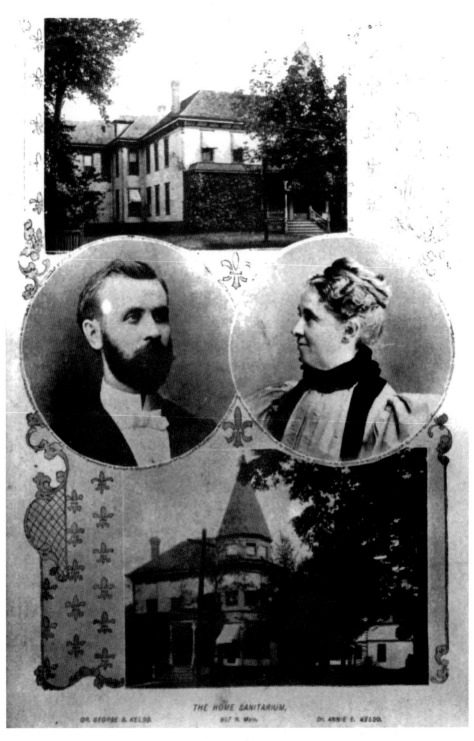

THE HOME SANITARIUM.

DR. GEORGE B. KELSO   807 N. Main   Dr. ANNIE E. KELSO

Drs. George and Annie Kelso's Home Sanitarium

Dr. Joseph Price Noble, president of the Medical Society in 1930, was an age contemporary of Dr. Young's. Born in 1868, he graduated from Northwestern University Medical School in 1893. At that time, the school had "only three full-time men on its staff: the registrar, janitor, and professor of chemistry."[18] In 1910, Abraham Flexner had called Chicago "the plague spot of the country" with regard to the quality of medical education it offered. While he indicated that Northwestern, Rush and the College of Physicians and Surgeons, a proprietary school which joined the University of Illinois in 1913, were nationally competitive, they were merely the best of a bad lot. Only after 1911 did Northwestern require applicants to have two years of college preparation before beginning medical training.[19]

Dr. Daniel D. Raber, born in 1878 and president of the McLean County Medical Society in 1940, received his medical diploma from Bennett Medical College of Eclectic Medicine and Surgery in 1908, two years before the school merged with several other colleges to form the medical department of Loyola University.[20] Dr. Raber practiced as a general practitioner, was on the staffs of St. Joseph's, Mennonite and Brokaw hospitals, and held teaching positions in the nursing schools of Brokaw and St. Joseph's hospitals.

Despite the longevity of traditional preparation for medical practice, however, change was coming. For example, Dr. Frank Deneen, president of the McLean County Medical Society in 1927, represented a newer generation of physicians. Born in 1890, he received his undergraduate education at Illinois Wesleyan University and the University of Chicago. He received his M.D. degree from Northwestern University Medical School in 1915, then took internships at St. Louis City Hospital and the Children's Free Hospital in Detroit, Michigan. Dr. Deneen specialized in internal medicine; his preparation for medical practice was typical for physicians trained after 1910. It remains typical of physicians practicing in McLean County in the second half of the twentieth century.

Practitioners' Perspectives

This study benefits greatly from the oral history interviews provided by six physicians and one dentist.[21] All but one of these professionals practiced in McLean County; four of them located in Bloomington. One physician, Dr. Welch, practiced in Cuba, Illinois, a small community in Fulton County. His experience, together with that of Dr. Boon of Danvers, Dr. Oyer of Chenoa, and Dr. Shinall, who practiced in Gibson City during the mid-1930s, provides information about rural practice.

Table 1: Physicians and Dentists

Name	Year of birth	Occupation	Professional school	Location of practice
Harold Shinall	1909	Physician (Radiologist)	University of Illinois	Gibson City Bloomington
James Welch	1915	Physician (GP)	St. Louis University	Cuba
Loren Boon	1917	Physician (GP)	University of Illinois	Danvers
W.L. Dillman	1920	Dentist	University of Illinois	Bloomington
Russell Oyer	1920	Physician (GP)	University of Illinois	Chenoa
Paul Theobald	1922	Physician (GP)	University of Illinois	Bloomington
Albert VanNess	1926	Physician (Internist)	Indiana University	Bloomington

To some extent, the practitioners interviewed represent continuity in professional health care. All of them were trained after the reform of medical education. Thus, they had pre-medical undergraduate university educations before embarking on four-year professional training programs. They all took internships; medical specialists completed residencies. These practitioners began their careers after the establishment of bio-medical science as the single theory dominating medical practice and after professional medicine had achieved a legally protected monopoly over the provision of medical care. Thus, they expected and assumed the physician's enormous mid-twentieth-century position of authority and were more likely to remark on the relatively recent perceived decline in that authority than to marvel at how popular perceptions of the physician's expertise grew during their years in practice.

Nonetheless, the practitioners interviewed have also seen tremendous changes in the practice of medicine. Their lives span the transition from a profession dominated by general practitioners to one led by specialists. They have witnessed the shift, more dramatic in rural than urban areas in the mid-twentieth century, from practice largely conducted in patients' homes to institutionally-based health care. They have also experienced a transformation in medical economics from the relatively simple individual payment (or barter) for services rendered to the inflation of medical costs which brought health insurance with it.

The interview respondents have also participated in dramatic changes in the efficacy of medical interventions. Those trained before the 1940s experienced the impact on medical and surgical practice of the introduction of antibiotics. All of the practitioners interviewed became accustomed to using an increasing range of medical technologies which enhanced diagnostic, monitoring and therapeutic processes. They also experienced the inflation of patient's expectations which both increased the status and incomes of physicians and stimulated the growth in malpractice litigation after the 1960s.

The Decision to Become a Doctor

By the second quarter of the twentieth century when most of the practitioners interviewed were making career decisions, medicine was a well established profession — like law or the ministry, a respectable, high-status occupation. However, it was by no means an easy option. W.L. Dillman, born in 1920, who had intended to go into medicine but eventually opted for dentistry, based his career choice on his father's experience of medical practice in Louisville, Kentucky. He remembered:

> He [my father] worked so hard. Have you ever seen any of these wall telephones with a crank on the side and you take the receiver off the other side? I can hear that thing ringing in the night. . . . They didn't have "no night calls" or "no house calls" in those days. He had house calls, night calls; I've gone with him down the railroad tracks at night in the winter time after a train would go through to clear a path in the snow. I'd walk and carry his medical bag and we'd walk down the tracks somewhere, and maybe someone would meet us with a wagon. I'd go to sleep in the kitchen, and maybe he'd deliver a child or something.[22]

Dillman made the decision to become a dentist when his father died just as he was finishing his pre-medical education.

Dr. Dillman's experience was apparently typical for sons of physicians, many of whom grew up carrying medical equipment and visiting patients' homes. However, in contrast to his decision, many of these men followed in their father's footsteps. Indeed, in 1954 the *Biographical History of the McLean County Medical Society* listed no fewer than 17 sons of physician parents among their members.[23] Three of the seven practitioners interviewed for this study were doctors' sons whose recollections extend backward to conditions of practice which had changed by the time they joined the profession. This lore influenced their decisions to become physicians. Like W.L. Dillman, James Welch, the son and grandson of doctors who, like himself, practiced for many years in Cuba, Illinois, also remembered traveling with his father when he made house calls, saying "I guess that's the way I got interested."[24]

Like other respondents, Welch was impressed by the special status of physicians in small towns. During the 1919 flu epidemic, he recalled:

> Every doctor in the county was sick except two, and Dad was one of them. He'd see his patients and then at night he would drive to Canton and just go around and knock on the doors, "Do you need a doctor?" one door to the next. Well, in those days the car didn't have anti-freeze, and if you stopped you had to leave the motor running or drain her out and refill her again. Well, . . . he went down checking in the square and parked his car. He wanted some medicine and he wanted to get a cigar, so he left the motor running. But Canton had just passed an ordinance. It was a high crime misdemeanor to leave the motor running. Some of these cars would take off! So he came out, and here were a couple of cops. He left his motor running and they caught him. They were taking him down the street, fussing him all the way, "You're going to the pokey!" So as they were going along, this one cop said, "Who are you anyway?" "Well," he says, "I'm Dr. Welch from Cuba." And they stopped and they said, "You the one that's been going around town?" They were really frightened! They said, "Do you know that they would lynch us, the townspeople would, if they knew we arrested you?" So they got him back, got his car going, and sent him home. Dad always laughed at how frightened those policemen were."[25]

Loren Boon, born in 1917, was also the son of a doctor. He grew up expecting to go into medicine. He remembered that:

> I kind of liked science and things like that. And . . . I kind of thought that [medicine] would be the place to go. . . . I remember one incident. . . in high school. . . they were having a ball game and a man got hit in the head. . . and had

some bleeding or something. Somebody asked me if that didn't bother me, and I said, "Nope." "You must gonna be a doctor then." No, I didn't faint or anything.[26]

Albert VanNess, born in 1926, did not come from a medical family; his father worked for State Farm and his mother worked as a receptionist in a doctor's office. However, he grew up around physicians. "My mother was involved with medicine and . . . I knew doctors. . . . I met them through going up to the Gresheim Building to see my mother." He remembered admiring doctors:

> I was brought up that my folks taught me . . . and I don't recollect them talking about money. It was. . . that doctors are honored, revered people who are well educated. I can still remember Howard Sloan telling me one Christmas when I was home from the navy, "The interesting thing is that . . . the vocabulary of a physician is five times that of the average person."[27]

Born in 1909, Harold Shinall also said that he "admired several doctors, and just sort of approved of them. . . . I was impressed that even though they didn't have antibiotics they seemed to be able to make you well again." He had had diphtheria as a child and was treated with "shots of antitoxin." He had great respect for the doctor who cared for his family, and viewed physicians as effective and powerful in the struggle against disease. Further examining his reasons for going into medicine, Shinall said, "I would like to be able to reduce it to helping people, but I don't know that that was primarily the thing in those days. I think it was part of it. I liked to see the favorable outcomes I had observed."[28] Thus, several of the physicians interviewed went into medicine partly because of role models identified during childhood.

Some respondents chose medicine because of its dramatic image. Born in 1920, Russell Oyer grew up on a farm. He recalled visiting his sister, who was eight years older than himself, during her training at Mennonite School of Nursing:

> She would take me to the hospital and the floors would be polished and you would . . . have those smells of ether and that sort of stuff. . . . The nurses walking up and down in their stiffly starched uniforms . . . taking care of people. I think maybe that was the early kind of fantasy. . . about medicine that sort of grew and impressed me, I guess. It

continued. When I started at Bluffton [College], I decided to take a few medicine courses.[29]

Finally, in some cases medicine was simply the natural career option for a bright young man. Paul Theobald, born in 1922, did not remember making a definite decision to go into medicine:

> I never planned on being a doctor until the day I graduated and thought, "that's it." I used to have a lot of infections as a kid, and everyone kept saying, "Oh, you ought to be a doctor and save some money." It never sunk into me, and basically I didn't make a decision, but it just seemed that I kept going. Pre-medicine, [I] still wasn't sure I wanted to go to medical school, but when I finished, it was like, "Well, I got to go to medical school. . . ." It was just one of those things: I went along until finally I graduated and I thought, "Well, I'm a doctor."[30]

Economic considerations were not significant in respondents' decisions to go into medicine. Of course, several interviewees were formulating their career aspirations during the Depression of the 1930s. As one local historian points out, "Doctors were its victims as was almost everyone else. Some lost their savings in the ruin of the stock market. Many of these succeeded in retrieving these losses by continuing their hard work."[31] Doctors did not earn as much during the Depression as they had in earlier years. James Welch remembered that during the 1930s:

> The banks were all closed. . . [My father] He'd go on a house call and he'd come back with a basket of turnips or chickens or eggs, or what-not. I was with him one day when we went on a call. There was this farmer who was bemoaning, and farmers were about ready to revolt, and Dad said, "Now, look here John. You got your chickens and your eggs, and your hogs. You got this garden." He outlined all the things, you know. He said, "You're not too bad." He [the farmer] said, "Doc, I'll tell you, you come back in a year and you'll see the fattest, nakedest farmer you ever saw!"[32]

Thus, status and the perceived drama of medical practice were more important factors than prospective incomes in motivating

young men to go into medicine during the period under consideration.

Medical Education

Although changes in medical education came quickly during the early years of the twentieth century, practitioners interviewed for this study remembered both earlier types of preparation for practice and resistance on the part of established physicians and patients to the innovations introduced by young doctors.
James Welch's father began practicing in Cuba, Illinois, in about
1909 after having taken post-graduate training at a hospital in
Minneapolis:

> When he came back. . . he was one of the first in his trade
> in aseptic surgery. . . . A lot of the old-timers were pretty
> skeptical of this new-fangled stuff. A lot of deliveries were
> done at home then. . . . He came back to his home town
> here and he insisted on wearing rubber gloves and boiling
> his instruments. At that time, they used lard. Can you
> imagine that? . . . These women thought if they greased
> themselves with lard it would make the baby come out eas-
> ier. It don't know what it did about that, but it sure
> increased infection. . . . So the talk went around among the
> ladies that he was pretty persnickety and he didn't want to
> get his hands dirty![33]

Such young physicians spearheaded the trend in favor of innova-
tive techniques which eventually became conventional even among
older practitioners.

The doctors interviewed for this study followed the pattern
established as standard after publication of the Flexner Report in
1910. They finished high school, then did university pre-medical
preparation before going to medical school. Not all interviewees
took undergraduate degrees. Harold Shinall spent only three
years at the University of Illinois in Champaign-Urbana (1927-
1930) before starting medical school at the University of Illinois in
Chicago. He explained, "At that time you could go on at the end of
three years to medical school if your grades were okay."[34] While it
became increasingly common for pre-medical students to finish
bachelor's degrees during the 1930s, the advent of World War II
temporarily shortened medical education. Loren Boon remembered spending two years at the University of Illinois in

Champaign before going to the University of Illinois's medical school in Chicago. He received his M.D. in 1942.[35] Russell Oyer, who went to medical school in the early 1940s, said, "At that time, still during the national emergency of World War II, at the medical school you did three academic years. You did four academic years in three calendar years. You went to school all the time."[36]

In contrast to today's aspiring physicians who are faced with the daunting challenge of raising huge sums to pay for their medical educations, doctors trained before 1950 reported that tuition charges were low, and that expense, although important, was not a barrier to obtaining university and medical educations. James Welch took his bachelor's degree at Knox College, a private school which was comparatively expensive by contemporary standards. He remembered paying $150-200 per semester beginning in 1933, and that his father borrowed money to send him to school. However, he was able to give up his part-time job as a busboy in a cafeteria in order to "devote myself to football" fairly early in his college career.[37]

Dr. Shinall, whose father, the only wage earner in the home, was an insurance agent, said that he chose the University of Illinois' undergraduate program for financial reasons:

> *Interviewer*: Did you ever consider going anywhere else?
> *Respondent*: I didn't have the money. That [U. of I.] was
> only 32 miles away from Danville. My first year I worked
> while going to school. I would go home on weekends, hitch-
> hiked, and I would work in that Penney's store on
> Saturdays. My sophomore year I got a job as a waiter on
> the campus. The third year I was in a pre-medical fraterni-
> ty and was named the treasurer and if you had that job as
> sort of a manager, you got your room and board provided.[38]

At $25 per semester, undergraduate tuition was less of a challenge than maintenance. Shinall obtained a scholarship through the state legislature when he started medical school in 1930. "You'll be shattered to think of how little it was in those days. . . . The tuition at the medical school was $100 per semester. But a dollar was worth more then too, so it's relative."[39]

Paul Theobald, whose father had died when he was a child, had a partial scholarship to attend Illinois Wesleyan University as an undergraduate. In addition, he worked part-time jobs:

> Starting in high school days I was a *Pantagraph* carrier,

and I carried papers up through the Freshman year at Illinois Wesleyan, and I was an usher at the Irvin Theater and became Assistant Manager over at the Castle Theater, and then during the war years I worked at Eureka Williams as a First Aid Attendant on the night shift between 11 at night and 7 in the morning. At the same time I attended Illinois Wesleyan, carried a full course, and also had a date every night. I was busy.[40]

Russell Oyer's father was a tenant farmer who "farmed with horses ." He remembered about his family's economic situation:

We didn't have indoor plumbing at all during my growing up. There was no running water inside, no indoor toilet. A very simple home. We were really poor. Then the Depression hit, of course, the crash in 1929 and the early years of the 1930s. But I don't think you thought so much about that in those days because everyone else was sort of in the same boat. . . . We always had enough to eat, and we had a house to live in. But there was no money.[41]

He got a small scholarship and borrowed money to attend Bluffton College in Ohio for undergraduate school:

I was able to borrow some money, my sister helped me quite a bit, and my mother helped a little bit during college, but I also borrowed some money from a couple of relatives and some friends for college expenses. In those days, of course, college expenses were small, but it was a lot of money in those days.[42]

A number of respondents received all or part of their medical training courtesy of the armed forces or the GI Bill. Dr. Oyer borrowed money for medical school and equipment:

I was able to borrow some money and I started to school. I can't remember what we paid at the apartment. I don't think our room cost a great deal. I don't know what tuition was. . . . It seems to me that several hundred dollars might have been tuition. I remember I bought a microscope from A.S. Alo. . . . You could buy a binocular scope for $7.50 per month. . . . I finally got that paid off.[43]

His internship, however, was paid for by the military:

> The class was about 180 with five or six women. . . .
> Practically all of the males went to either the Navy pro-
> gram or the Army Specialized Training Program which
> were professional programs paid for by the government. . . .
> If you wanted to stay out of the draft, you had to sign up for
> Second Lieutenant status in the Reserves. Then you were
> permitted to finish medical school and in exchange for that
> you were committed then to two years of service after you
> graduated. You went from internship then directly to an
> assignment.[44]

After graduating from high school in 1944, Albert VanNess was drafted into the Navy which sent him to John Carroll University in Cleveland, Ohio:

> In the so-called Navy B-12 Program. . . you got $21 a
> month, room, board, and you went to school. . . . I was in
> John Carroll for 17 months and I had almost 90 hours
> when I left there. . . . I was thinking about medicine
> and . . .that was fortified by my experience at John Carroll.
> At John Carroll, they really taught you how to study. If you
> didn't cooperate with that, you found yourself in Great
> Lakes one week and about six weeks later out in the
> Pacific.[45]

After the war ended, the GI Bill supported the rest of VanNess's undergraduate education and medical training at Indiana University.

None of the interview respondents appear to have been worried about admission to medical school. In 1930, according to Harold Shinall, "The competition was there. You had to maintain a 3.5 to be eligible to go to med school. That would be one-half Bs and one- half Cs as they listed it then."[46] However, competition increased dramatically after World War II. By the time Albert VanNess finished his bachelor's degree in 1946, entrance to medical school was more competitive because of war-time interruptions to professional educations, large numbers of returning servicemen, and GI Bill support for the college educations of many who might not otherwise have thought medical training within their means:

> There were 5,000 applications [to Indiana University
> Medical School] and 141 were accepted. 100 went to
> Indianapolis [for the final three years of training].
> Eventually, though, I think 102 or 103 graduated, because
> in those years at least two to four medical students per
> class had to drop out because of tuberculosis or some ill-
> ness. . . .
> *Interviewer*: What would have been the make-up of your
> class? How many women were there?
> *Respondent*: Two. . . . Two out of 100. Two blacks. At the
> end of our sophomore year, Indiana always took two people
> from Mississippi, and two people from Alabama in the clinic
> years because those schools were two-year schools at the
> time. . . . We had two foreign students. . . . The class aver-
> age age was 27. . . . Some fellows in our class had started
> out in night school in the '30s and working and trying to get
> their pre-med together so they could eventually go to med-
> ical school. Some of those fellows got drafted. . . . One fel-
> low was 44 or 45, who had been the Dean of Men at Butler
> University before the war. But see, the GI Bill of Rights
> changed all that. . . . It was a varied and sundry group of
> people. . . .[47]

Other practitioners also remembered that their medical school
classes were largely white and male, although some were educated
with a few more women. Harold Shinall said:

> In fact, my lab partner was a woman. . . . She later became
> a pediatrician in Danville. I think it was only a small num-
> ber, about one-half dozen [women in the class]. My grand-
> daughter [who recently began medical school] has about
> one-third. So that's been a big change.[48]

Dr. Shinall indicated that, while most of his medical colleagues
were men, a somewhat older medical generation actually included
more women. During his medical training he had a part-time job
working on the switchboard at the Women's and Children's
Hospital which had "almost entirely women on the staff. . . There
were some prominent women surgeons and I think they were pretty self sufficient. Occasionally they would have some man come in
as a patient, but I don't think they really had any men listed on
staff."[49]

All physicians interviewed for this study received very similar training. The oldest respondent, Harold Shinall, who began his professional training in 1928, described the University of Illinois' medical school curriculum as follows:

> The medical training was four years. They described the first two years as pre-clinical and the second two years as clinical because the first two years you had anatomy, histology, endocrinology, neurology, and all that, with microscopic and gross anatomy, physiology, and you don't have a stethoscope. The latter part of your second year you continue on pre-clinical courses. You get into a little surgical instruction in classroom and so forth. You started in on physical diagnosis at that time and you got a stethoscope. Then the last two years you still continued courses in surgery and internal medicine and the other little smaller practices, but in addition to that, there were a lot of visits to the operating room and outpatient clinics and deliveries.[50]

At the younger end, Russell Oyer, trained in the 1940s, remembered that his pre-clinical courses were also concentrated during the first two years of medical school, although he participated in what was then a novel attempt to integrate the scientific preparation for medical practice:

> Dr. Otto Kentmeyer had the vision that medicine ought to be well correlated so that really students would study, not human anatomy, histology, genetics, . . . chemistry, but they would study medicine. . . . So he wrote his own laboratory textbook on the human anatomy which did, indeed, correlate and incorporate, integrate the gross anatomy, histology; so actually you were in the lab dissecting part of the time, studying histology part of the time, you know, it was really an attempt to correlate the whole approach to human medicine. . . . I think patient contact started, well, physical diagnosis I think was taught in the second year. You started getting some patients after that, but basically clinical contact was the Junior year.[51]

Albert VanNess remembered that his first year of medical training, which was conducted on the Bloomington campus of Indiana University, was made deliberately difficult in order to reduce from 141 to 100 the number of students who would continue their training at the medical school campus in Indianapolis:

> It was a very nerve-wracking year. They really put the
> pressure on you. They literally drove some people right out
> of there that didn't seem to have what it takes. . . . It was-
> n't nearly as difficult as I thought it was going to be to
> make the Indianapolis cut because it [the first year] was
> terrible on some people.[52]

W.L. Dillman, the dentist interviewed for this study,
remembered that his training was similar to that taken by medical students:

> In those days we had a lot of the same courses and instruc-
> tors that the medical students did. We were right across
> the street from Cook County Hospital. We'd go over and
> watch the operations and a lot of the work. . . . Some of the
> fellows did not see why we should have to work on cadav-
> ers, go to autopsies, until a professor finally explained to us
> how each part of the body can affect another part of the
> body. We were taught to observe any pathology in any way.
> Why do you think they look down your throat and say,
> "Stick out your tongue?" That's one of the first places you
> look for pathology.[53]

Clinical training, which occurred during the last two years
of medical school and continued during internships and residencies, involved exposure to a range of medical conditions, introduction to therapeutic techniques, and progressive degrees of responsibility taken by the student. It was in this area that the urban
locations of mid-twentieth-century medical schools made their
most significant contributions to medical training, since large city
populations provided inexhaustible material for observation and
practice. Many of the "guinea-pigs" for medical students' early
diagnostic and therapeutic efforts were drawn from among the
urban poor, who went to public hospitals and dispensaries, also
used for teaching purposes, because they could not afford the fees
of private facilities.

In particular, most physicians interviewed for this study
remembered attending home deliveries, which were arranged
through the hospitals. Dr. VanNess recalled the social conditions
in Indianapolis in the years immediately following World War II:

In those days they had no way to get all the women into the hospital to give birth. So if a woman had one . . . uneventful birth, when she got pregnant the second time, she went on the outdoor service, and the hospital gave you an automobile, two students, a medical bag, and they . . . went out and delivered the child in the home. . . . I could fill up three tapes about what happened on that because, of course, you end up delivering prostitutes and people living in garages. See, during the war, there was a tremendous movement of people into Indianapolis. . . . So there were a lot of people that were relatively destitute and there was no housing for them, and nobody was building anything during the war. So people'd fix up their garages and people would move into their garage and pay rent for this and have no sanitation.[54]

James Welch had similar memories of St. Louis during the 1930s:

Well, in our senior year, after we had lectures and been over at the university hospital in OB and so forth, we were sent out in groups of three. . . into the . . . tenements, the district along the river, you know, and worked with the poor. . . . We had delivered babies in the hospital, but when we had to go out by ourselves, we were three, one to give the anesthesia, one to take care of the baby (these were home deliveries) and one to deliver the baby. And then they had residents, nurses, in these vans that went around and kept close contact, you know. . . . We went to this first one and . . . we had a resident. He thought all medical students were idiots, which is probably true. . . . We went in this one, this was a big lady. She was lying on a feather tick. . . . We came in like gang busters, you know. All of us scared to death. She laughed at us all the way through everything. Which didn't help. . . . But anyway, the baby was precipitated just as we came in the door. In other words, baby, placenta, everything came out —- whoosh! She'd had eleven children! . . . But there was a big rip in this old feather tick. And it all went down. We were really frightened then because we thought the baby [would smother]. We go to get him out. We cut the cord, took him to the kitchen, and he was covered with vernix, you know, the cold cream-like stuff. . . . And we were standing there looking at him, and I swear, maybe it's exaggerated now, but he was covered with feathers from head to toe. . . . Just then this resident walked in the back door of the kitchen. And he stared. He said, "What are you goddamn idiots doing now?!" This one idiot said, "Well, we're picking the feathers off the baby!"[55]

All of the practitioners interviewed did internships. Harold Shinall explained:

> The U. of I., in those days, along with two other medical schools in the Midwest, did not actually give you your M.D. degree until the completion of your internship. Theoretically, you couldn't be called a doctor yet, but at the graduation ceremony, we were handed a little certificate that said we had completed the four years of medical training. . . .

Most respondents were married by this point in their training. The pattern was for wives to continue working while husbands worked demanding call schedules and earned nominal stipends of between ten and twenty-five dollars a month. Russell Oyer remembered:

> Each of us had a room at the hospital where we stayed when we were on call. . . . I think every three or four nights I was in the hospital . . . .
> *Interviewer*: What were those days like? What was an on-call day?
> *Respondent*: Well, history and physical on new patients and a conference with the attending physician. You would follow, you'd make rounds with the attending physician. You'd write a few orders. Not all orders. You did everything in consultation with the attending physician. You did an obstetrical kind of thing, and you did a medical thing, and you did a surgical thing. Surgery, then you'd be scrubbing for cases that you were on.[57]

Albert VanNess said of his internship at the University of Chicago:

> It was forever!. . . It was around the clock, weekends, holidays, the whole business. You were just on call every other day and worked every day of course for 12 hours. It was brutal. . . . We'd have some services that have 30 or 40 people on them, and you'd run that by yourself and most of the attendants up there would just turn you loose if they didn't

think you needed much supervision. You'd get on the hematology service, and you'd give 25 transfusions in the morning and admit people in the afternoon and scrub and do bone marrows.[58]

Several respondents did their internships during military service.

Both World War II and family responsibilities affected respondents' decisions about whether to take a residency to qualify as a specialist. Doctors Welch, Boon and Oyer had considered specializing in internal medicine. James Welch explained that military service interrupted his plans; when he finished his four-year army service, he went into practice with his father in order to support his family.[59] Loren Boon recalled:

> I went right from internship and got married. I thought I was going to come back for residency there at Ravenswood Hospital in Chicago. I came back from getting married, a honeymoon, and there was a . . . letter in a brown envelope telling me to report for service on July 1st.[60]

When he finished military service, he finished one year of general residency at Milwaukee Hospital. Then, in 1947, he went into practice, where he was able to develop an informal specialty in anesthesiology.

Russell Oyer remembered:

> When I was about ready to be . . . separated from the services, I guess I was really interested in internal medicine and did check out at least a couple places in Chicago. . . .. At that point, there was a lot of competition for the best spots in residency because of everybody getting out of the service at that time [1946]. . . . I did think about that and retrospectively, as I have thought about my career, I think I would have been much happier in a specialty practice. . . . But our three kids came along and I started deferring decisions about getting going with training. . . .[61]

By the 1940s, the trend toward specialization was already pronounced. Indeed, Harold Shinall, who worked as a general practitioner during the 1930s, decided to undertake a residency in radiology in 1940. He explained:

I put an x-ray machine in my office. . . . Early on, I realized my shortcomings because I would be saying things that I wasn't sure of. I had a brother-in-law who was a radiologist, practicing in East St. Louis. The cases I was not sure about, I would send him the films for interpretation. I visited him a few times and decided that maybe I'd like to do that. He knew the doctor that was in charge at the city hospital, and so he arranged for me to go down for an interview. . . . I was there at the city hospital for two years and then I went into the military. I was associated with the army general hospital. When I finished up my period of time, I was able to apply for the board examination.[62]

Shinall decided to specialize, in part, because of the lack of hospital facilities in Gibson City where he had practiced as a GP. However, he reflected that his experience in general practice "helped me after I got established because I was able to handle patients a little bit better than people who had not had that prior experience."[63]

Albert VanNess decided to specialize in internal medicine during his internship at the University of Chicago:

I was interested in everything. I started out thinking I was going to become an ENT man, but that I'm sure was because of Dr. Watkins' influence and my mother working for him. But I realized I didn't like that. Then I thought of some other things, even OB/GYN. And then, later on in my internship, when you had to start scrubbing up and being there for hours, then I lost enthusiasm for surgical procedures and that's when I began to think about medicine.[64]

After spending two years in military service during the Korean War, he finished his residency at the University of Chicago between 1954 and 1957.

Going Into Practice

Most of the physicians interviewed for this study located where they did because of personal contacts. James Welch went into practice with his father in Cuba, Illinois. Paul Theobald worked briefly with a physician in a resort area in Wisconsin. Then:

We went out to California and I looked things over out

there, and I thought we had no money and I knew this was no place for a practitioner because when hard times come we'd be hit. So. . . we decided we would come back to Bloomington where we knew some people that if we needed some money we could borrow some.[65]

Albert VanNess also chose to practice in Bloomington because of social contacts, which were especially important to a new specialist, dependent on referrals:

We came to Bloomington for Max Stevenson's wedding . . . at the Country Club I think it was. . . . I got to talking to Ed Stevenson and at the time I knew that it was time for me to leave. I wanted to go to somewhere else than the University of Chicago. We had great training up there. It was wonderful and I had a good experience, but I wanted to move on and the ethnic neighborhoods were changing very rapidly. Judy was pregnant and we had two children. We were trying to decide what to do. Ed Stevenson was the one that persuaded me to come to Bloomington. . . . He said that he would fix me up. That we would kind of practice in parallel if I accepted, and that he would contribute to getting me off the ground.[66]

W.L. Dillman, who lived in Bloomington as a child, learned that the newly organized County Health Department was looking for a dentist at the time he finished his military service. He was employed by the Department for eight years, helping to set up the water fluoridation program in McLean County.[67]

Harold Shinall discovered an opening for a doctor in Gibson City through a friend who was practicing in Piper City:

We learned that there was an elderly physician in Gibson City who was suffering from cancer of the stomach and was not expected to live very long. I went to see him, and I took his office over. . . . During the remainder of his life, I had to pay him a certain percentage of what my income was. I took over his equipment; a lot of it was antiquated. He died within a year; so then I took over.[68]

Loren Boon had been raised in Washburn, Illinois, where his father had practiced medicine. He decided not to locate there because the community was positioned midway between the hospitals in Peoria and Spring Valley; thus, doctors did a great deal of traveling to visit hospitalized patients. However, he wanted to return to central Illinois, and selected Danvers, partly because residents used only the hospitals in Bloomington.[69]

Physicians settling in rural communities during the early twentieth century had working conditions which changed radically by the end of their careers. For one thing, in those years there were many more doctors. When Dr. Welch's father began practicing in Cuba in 1908 or 1909, there were seven doctors serving a population of fewer than 2,000 residents.[70] Although they maintained offices and visited patients in accessible hospitals, the majority of their time was spent visiting patients in their own homes, sometimes more than once a day. In communities without hospitals, the sick were cared for under the most comfortable circumstances that could be provided. Dr. Welch recalled a family story:

> The train pulled in down here and they took a woman off the train that was deathly sick. Here was the tracks and here was this old hotel there, and they put her in the hotel. They called Dad to see her. She was in really bad shape. My parents had just gotten married. My mother was only 18. She [the patient] had pneumonia. Dad found an empyema, you know. . . [a] pocket of pus. . . . She [Mother] hadn't had any medical experience or anything, but he wanted to get a tube in to get that pus out of there. So he had her [Mother] give the anesthesia. With ether, you know. . . . And of course, she [Mother] was scared to death about that. They got her [patient] asleep and Dad had this tube ready to go in. He just made this incision in the thorax and the pus was everywhere. Just drenched my mother; vile smelling! . . . They got that tube in her and a stitch or two in her. She was at death's door for a long time. He took care of her. Finally she began to mend and she told Dad many times, "I don't have any money." She'd always say, "But I won't forget you." Dad thought, well. . . . So, somehow she got enough money to get a train ticket somewhere out west. Got on the train one day and took off. Now that would have been in 1915 or 1916. I came back here in 1946. . . . I was with him in the post office one day and he got this package. It was a wad of money that would choke a horse.
> *Interviewer*: My goodness! From that woman?
> *Respondent*: Yeah.[71]

Physicians beginning practice in the 1930s were already experiencing the trend in favor of institutionally-based medical care which began in the early years of the century. Physician-patient ratios changed as office and hospital practice became increasingly common and automobile travel became easier. Nonetheless, Dr. Shinall recalled that when he started practicing in Gibson City in 1935, there were three other doctors working there. At that time, the community had a population of 2,200, and physicians treated many patients who lived in the surrounding rural area. Since house calls were still usual, physicians had plenty to do. Shinall said, "I remember, I went in to see one of them [local doctors] before I started, and he said, 'I don't care how well you do here, just so I keep my share.'"[72]

Dr. Shinall took over an established physician's office, so he was spared the expense of building and decorating a new office. However, he also had to deal with conditions which seemed old-fashioned even at the time:

> Well, he had a hard coal stove in the office. After the winter of '35/'36, they still speak of how cold it was, and I had to lug the coal up from the back outside, up the steps to the office and bank it at night to keep it warm enough. Then I could just stoke it up a little bit in the morning. There was a waiting room and a larger room.[73]

Dr. Shinall dispensed medications himself. He also administered ultraviolet treatment and eventually had a diathermy machine. He divided his time between making house calls, many to patients some miles distant from town; visiting patients hospitalized in Bloomington and Paxton; and seeing patients in his office.

To some extent, Shinall inherited his clientele from the physician whose practice he took over. He was also eager to develop a good reputation among patients so that word of mouth would bring him new customers. He said, "In those days physicians didn't place ads. That was sort of frowned upon and so you did the best that you can as far as work is concerned and let that speak for itself." He encountered the full range of health problems, from farm injuries, to contagious diseases, to childbirth:

> *Interviewer*: What kinds of things were you mainly dealing with?
> *Respondent*: The skin and its contents, I guess. Well, there were a lot of infections in those days, and we did not have antibiotics. So a lot of things that are controlled in a brief

period with antibiotics now had complications a lot of times. . . . You don't hear about a quinsy throat or a pair of tonsillar abscesses any more, but I had a few of those. A lot of infectious diseases I think would make up a lot of my clients.[74]

James Welch also remembered dealing with illnesses not commonly encountered today. The first patient he treated when he began practicing in 1946 had typhoid fever. He also remembered:

Well, I had this cousin. . . . He was a surgeon, a good surgeon. Dad and I were up there making rounds with him one morning at the hospital and he says, "You know, I've got this patient with the strangest damn rash, and I can't diagnose it." Well, let's go take a look at it." We went in, "Oh, my God!" he said. We went outside, and he [cousin] said, "What's the matter?" He [father] says, "It's small pox.". . . . They had never seen it.[75]

It was usual for doctors to make house calls. Shinall recalled:

You had to have a car because you had a lot of calls in the country in those days. House calls are not too prevalent these days. One reason is emergency rooms and so forth, but I've had people call me after a snow storm and say they planned to come in, but the snow was pretty deep, and wondered if I'd mind coming out! . . . I had a friend that was a patient. He and I went on some trips when we took shovels and were able to get to places they couldn't get through.[76]

The rural physician's schedule was grueling. Shinall remembered:

The doctors who were there when I went there were having evening office hours as well as daytime office hours, so I had office hours in the morning, daytime, and evening, but I tried to get as many of my office patients in the afternoon and evening because in the morning you could make calls. I came over here to see my patients if they were hospitalized in Bloomington. There was also a hospital about 15 miles to the east of Gibson City, Paxton, Illinois; they had a hospital there and I did use that some. Some days I'd drive here and Paxton both, which was about 100 miles. I had made on unusual days three or four trips to Bloomington. . . . Because you might be over here for a surgical case in the morning, have an accident case in the evening, and an OB case at night. You were late a lot of times.[77]

Shinall did not take appointments. Rather, he saw patients on a first come, first served basis. During the early years of his practice, his wife worked in his office; later, he hired a graduate from Mennonite Hospital Nursing School to serve as nurse, receptionist and records manager.

In the late 1930s, patients became increasingly accustomed to traveling to doctors' offices and hospitals for treatment. Younger physicians encouraged this trend, particularly for deliveries. According to Harold Shinall:

> I think when I first started over there about two [deliveries] out of three would be in the home. By the time I left, I was encouraging them to go to the hospital and I had reversed that so there were two out of three in the hospital. *Interviewer*: What was the reason that you encouraged them to go in; greater safety? *Respondent*: I think so. . . . I think we were becoming educated to the fact about that time that this was a good idea.[78]

By the time Loren Boon went into practice in 1947, while house calls were still common for rural practitioners, office practice and hospital deliveries were the rule:

> Especially out here, when people wanted a house call, why they were sick enough to need a house call. That was just not always the case . . . in a larger city. But, yeah, I was making house calls up until the time I retired. . . . There were fewer because of the good roads and they probably realized I was able to give them better treatment at the office . . . than with what I was carrying in my medical bag. I even made a few deliveries at home. Not too many, . . .because that changed during World War II. . . and I think more of them got used to going to the hospital.[79]

When Paul Theobald went into practice in Bloomington in 1953, urban medical practice focused on office consultations and hospital visits. Many physicians rented space in the downtown Gresheim, Peoples Bank, and Unity buildings. Theobald remembered:

> Jill [wife] saw Mr. Impson at the Unity Building and he had an office space which previously had been a dentist's office . . . . We rented the office from him, and Jill told him, "We don't have any money. If he doesn't make any money the first month, we won't be able to pay you." And he said, "I have no worry about that. He'll make a go of it. You just pay me the rent whenever you can." And so we hooked up the office and there was a salesman by the name of Robinson from Gibson City. Robbie came over to visit me. He'd heard I'd set up in practice, and told me I could have whatever equipment I wanted and I could pay it off no interest or anything. We got the office waiting-room furniture from chairs from the altar — big straight chairs that had been in the church there for years and years. . . . I hired a nurse who had been working for Dr. Ed Stevenson. He was going to have to let her go, and I told her that I might not be able to pay her at the end of the week because I didn't have any money at all. . . . Dr. Nord called me up (he's a second cousin of my wife's). Stan called and said, "Paul, I want to take a vacation. Would you take calls for me?" I said sure! And that's how I got started.

Theobald's schedule revolved around office and hospital patients:

> Most doctors took Thursday afternoon off, but I found out that I was so busy taking calls for the other doctors on Thursday that I changed my afternoon off to Wednesday and then I'd work Thursday afternoon. I'd go to the hospitals in the morning, and . . . I think I'd get in [to the office] around 10:00 in the morning and see patients from 10 to 12 and then I'd take lunch and be back from 1 til 5. And then I making hospital calls at all three hospitals: Brokaw, St. Joe, and Mennonite every morning and every evening. I would also have office calls on Saturday morning.

In 1955, Theobald was at the forefront of a developing trend for physicians to move out of the city center. He said:

> In fact, the first person who moved out. . . from downtown

was actually Dr. Parker, and he moved out about the same time I did. . . . I remember Reverend Loydall, minister at the First Baptist Church, . . . [who] was on the Planning Commission and he heard I was going to move out on East Oakland. He came to me one day and said, "Paul, don't move out. You will ruin your practice. You won't make it out there." Well, I went ahead and moved out and actually the first month I was out there my business doubled. My auditor, when he saw it he just said there'd been a lot of business. He told me not to think that moving out had anything to do with it. In the second month it went up three times and about the fourth month my auditor said, "Well, it's quite evident that the move did do you a lot of good." My business really went up when I moved out. . . . Well, uptown you'd see one member of a family. . . . When I moved out on East Oakland, they'd come out in the car and you'd see the whole family. There'd be five or six instead of just one person. . . . I though that had more to do with it than anything.[80]

Theobald also made house calls. However, as patients became increasingly mobile, office- and hospital-based practice became more feasible and physicians' time was organized more cost-effectively. At the height of his practice, Dr. Theobald remembered seeing "Upwards of 100 patients a day in my office."[81]

Professional Relationships

After World War II, medicine was increasingly specialized. Nonetheless, informal part-time specialties, common at the turn of the century, continued. For example, Loren Boon, was trained to administer anesthesia during his general residency at Milwaukee hospital. He recalled that when he started practice in 1947, "Here I was. . . before the hospitals had their own anesthesia schools . . . . All they had were about two or three nurse anesthetists and then one MD anesthesiologist . . . . So I got busy right away with that too."[82] In addition, general practitioners continued to deliver babies and often did their own surgery. Paul Theobald remembered, "I was assisting in surgery, I would say probably four days out of the week. And I was delivering as many babies as any of the obstetricians . . . in town."[83] However, a growing number of physicians was obtaining formal board certification to practice an increasing range of medical specialties.

Relationships between general practitioners and specialists were important to all concerned. GPs cultivated relationships with specialists to whom they routinely referred patients. Dr. Theobald recalled:

> [For] OB work I used Dr. O.H. Ball. Almost entirely until Dr. Calhoun came into town. Cal and I became very good friends, and a high percentage of my work went to Calhoun. Ball was just very busy, and although he was very courteous and treated me well, . . . Cal and I just became very close friends and I . . . referred a lot to him. With surgery, I used Dr. Wilbur Ball until Dr. John Trish came to town . . . . John and I became friends and so I started referring a lot of patients to John. . . . The medical problems . . . were referred to Dr. Ed Livingston, and then eventually to Owen [Deneen]. . . . Pediatrics? . . . I used Dew a lot. In fact, I don't remember using Dr. Cline. He was a pediatrician in town. I don't recall using him very much.[84]

Russell Oyer discussed the way he made referrals:

> I think that I had fairly good relationships with the people I referred to. In those days, you had basically general internists. The general internist was your primary source of referral and he was the person who saw the patient with you and was able to make suggestions. Then you had the surgeon. . . . You had dermatologists, and some allergists, and some endocrinologists, . . . and some neurologists. . . but basically the first source of referral was a general internist. . . . In OB, for example, . . . Jim Brown would help me a lot in OB. He's just a great guy and was able to help. . . . I tried never to refer the patient unless I had done a good deal of work-up. I always felt that I needed to send a letter of referral.[85]

Strong professional relationships were even more important to specialists than to general practitioners. When Harold Shinall began practicing radiology in Bloomington in 1946, he had the advantage of the relationships he had developed as a GP sending patients to Bloomington hospitals. During his search for a practice location:

> I made inquiry up here and found out that St. Joseph's had learned that I was looking. They invited me to come up. I said, "Well, I'd like to talk to the administrator at

Mennonite and if I can come to both places, I'll come." And that worked out. . . . They knew me and I knew the hospitals and people. That certainly didn't hurt a bit. . . . One of the older doctors who was here as I was leaving Gibson City, when I told him what I was going to do, he said, "Harold, you're making a mistake. That specialty is going to be out the window. Doctors are putting in their own [x-ray] equipment and they'll be taking care of it. You won't have anything to do." We, he didn't envision enough, of course — I didn't either at that time — how the use of radiology would be expanded.[86]

Albert VanNess indicated that, for a new specialist in town, the significant relationships were with both established specialists and general practitioners. Established specialists often asked younger practitioners to substitute for them for emergency room and weekend call. VanNess said:

In those days, there wasn't anybody in the emergency room and that [taking call] was part of the deal. The older doctors got the younger doctors to take [their call] . . . and that's where I first ran across Sly Goldburg and people like that. We'd meet in the emergency room. Because we were out there at night because people like Ed Stevenson and Bob Price and Ray Baxter, . . . their names were on the rotation call, but . . . if they could get a substitute, the substitute's name was out there. . . It was a heck of a good way to start up a practice, but you were spending your entire night at the emergency room.

General practitioners referred within stable networks:

So usually what happened was, as an internist you would tie onto a couple of practitioners and they didn't vary; they sent you the business. They didn't call in one of fourteen. . . . Even the nurses would call you up and say, "There's a patient of Dr. Stevenson's here in the emergency room and you ought to see it because it had this or that." I shouldn't say Dr. Stevenson, I should say . . . Ray Doud or Dr. Williams, or somebody from the country. You know, people that lived out in the country, the physicians out in the country, if one of their patients . . . [was] in the hospital emergency room and you were their known consultant, you just went over there. You didn't even bother them until the next morning. They didn't want to come in from Danvers or any place like that in the middle of the night.[87]

In early years, relationships between general practitioners and surgeons were supported by the custom of splitting fees. According to A. Edward Livingston, who practiced internal medicine in Bloomington between 1945 and 1985:

> It was customary for the referring doctor to assist the surgeon. He would be paid by the surgeon for this help directly from the money received by him from the patient. The referring doctor would not have to send a bill but would receive a contracted part of the fee charged, hence the term "split fee." In itself, this does not seem to be a grave problem, but the difficulty in this method of payment lay in the fact that the referring doctors had the opportunity of selling their surgical patients to the highest bidder, not necessarily the best qualified surgeon. The referring doctor acting as a paid assistant was often unable to perform any part of the operation involved and so would not be able to take over the procedure should the need arise. Frequently the surgeon would operate on the referred patient without actually examining the patient to determine if there was definite need for an operation.[88]

When accreditation of hospitals by the American College of Surgeons became dependent upon medical staffs agreeing to stop splitting fees in the early 1950s, there was local objection. While physicians on staff at Brokaw and Mennonite hospitals accepted the new requirement, St. Josephs' staff members refused to comply. "It was then announced to the staff by the governing body of the Order of St. Francis in Peoria that the staff was disbanded and all former members had to reapply. Acceptance of their applications hinged on their signatures to suitable documents. . . . Thusly was the split-fee situation resolved."[89]

In early years, general practitioners dominated medical practice in McLean County. However, after the late 1950s, the balance shifted to specialists. Paul Theobald commented, "I enjoyed practicing medicine. I got very discouraged with . . . all the changes. I don't think that I would become a general practitioner again because I think GPs are about at the bottom of the totem pole as far as anyone else is concerned. . . ." At one point in his career, he considered doing a residency in surgery. While he decided against this move, he continued to do a lot of surgery:

> I gradually worked up just on my own by assisting. I got to the place where I had major surgical privileges and that was fine up until, oh, probably ten years ago when some of the younger doctors in town started coming, and they had gone back to this where GPs shouldn't be in the surgical department. I had a good reputation, and Dr. Fish often said that he'd rather have me help him in surgery than anyone else and he would call me on a lot of cases. The new young doctors wouldn't call me to assist on any of the patients. You could just tell by their attitude that "surgery is no place for a general practitioner to be." Which wasn't true in the old days. That's changed.[90]

Some general practitioners felt that specialists' higher status was reflected in the ways physicians were treated by hospital staff members and nurses. Dr. Theobald was offended when a patient he had recommended for sterilization was admitted to Mennonite hospital on a Sunday afternoon, with the procedure scheduled for Monday morning. On Sunday evening he was informed by the sterilization committee, which was required to approve all such procedures, that:

> I couldn't do the sterilization Monday morning. I got a little irritated and I found out that one of the . . . obstetricians got permission to do a sterilization on a patient who did not have near the requirements that my patient did. And so it was very embarrassing for me. That made me mad. I was making my rounds a couple weeks later and I remember walking in on the second floor by the nurses desk. . . and I went up to the desk like doctors do. Most days the nurses would stand up at attention when the doctor came in. . . and say, "What can I do for you, doctor?" I went up there and the girl working right at the desk looked at me, looked back down, and kept writing. . . . I just stood there five or ten minutes and finally all the girls jumped up at attention. . . . I looked down the corridor and half way down the corridor was Dr. Crowley [a specialist] coming down it. That's why they stood up at attention. I went down, saw the nursing supervisor, and I told her, "No one has shown me any courtesy, but if they're going to show one doctor courtesy then they should show it to all of them." So

I got mad, figured I didn't need Mennonite, so I quit
Mennonite then. Then gradually I just went over to St.
Joe. I don't know why.... Well, the Sisters were very nice,
and I am Protestant, and it wasn't a religious factor or anything like that but it was just easier for me to get my work
done. I had such a high admission out there that they
catered after my business. I could get almost anything I
wanted done out there.[91]

For some years, specialists dominated hospital staffs. However,
many physicians commented that, as financial considerations
become more important, administrators began making the important decisions.

Professional relationships were fostered by local, state and
national medical societies, which were also central in helping
practitioners keep up-to-date in their knowledge of new theories
and procedures. Dr. Boon remembered:

Shortly. . . after I started here . . . the American Academy of
General Practice started, and so I joined it. . . . And I
was able to go to national meetings and Peoria, over at
Peoria they eventually . . . developed some post graduate
courses. . . that were held throughout the state. . . . So we
managed to keep up pretty well.[92]

In addition, membership in the local medical society was also
important for cultivation of referral and social networks.

Professional organizations were expected to police their
members — something that was never easy. County medical societies were mainly concerned with infringements of medical ethics.
Russell Oyer recalled:

I think it was very difficult to get a hold of things like that.
I do remember once, we had a doctor who was quite popular in Bloomington. . . . He was doing a lot of OB. . . . I
think he was doing more OB really than some of the obstetricians in town at that point, but he also gave some anesthesia. The Medical Society at one point. . . wrote a letter
to him critical of his [decisions]. . . . Complaints had come
that his nurses were making decisions. They were seeing
the patient and giving medication and he was not seeing
the patient. He was an extremely busy guy. Then I
remember another physician who was turned in once for

advertising because he was doing something that seemed to the society as advertising.[93]

Physicians tended to handle privately issues of competence, supervising the hospital orders of an aging doctor whose judgment was suspect. According to Dr. Livingston:

> When a distinguished staff members suffered from a decline in his ability to direct the care of his patients, attempts were made to have him relinquish his practice, but this was almost always futile. So two charts were kept on his hospital admissions, unknown to him. A volunteer staff member would attend his patients to render the necessary care.

Hospital staff physicians also sanctioned members; privileges could be restricted or suspended in the case of doctors who were substance abusers or simply inept. [94]

Medical Economics

None of the practitioners interviewed expected physicians' incomes to increase as they did in the second half of the twentieth century. Their earnings expectations were low, as were fees in their early years of practice. Harold Shinall remembered that in 1935, "We attempted to keep a fee schedule and in the county and in the City of Gibson, our house calls were $3, office visits were $1.50, and calls in the country were $5.... Deliveries were $25."[95] Twenty years later, Russell Oyer's fees were similar:

> I came in 1954. I took everybody, whether they could pay or not. I didn't ask anybody about any credit things. And, of course, not so many people had insurance at that time either. You just took everybody, whether they paid or not. I started off with office calls at $3. We were delivering babies in Ohio for $35 and driving 10 miles to the hospital. I think I started with a fee of $50 here. I'm not sure, surgeons here got around $50-60. And of course here you drove 25 miles to the hospital.... I grew up in the Depression years and we had no money. I always had a lot of problem with fees and charging people to do things.

In his first month in practice, he earned $400.[96]

Even in those early years, specialists earned considerably

more than general practitioners. Albert VanNess recalls that in his first year of practice, 1958, he "netted somewhere between $10,000 and $12,000."[97] Nonetheless, this was a far cry from the sums newly qualified specialists earned in the last quarter of the century.

Physicians interviewed for this study were in mid-career when Medicare and Medicaid were introduced in the 1960s. Dr. Theobald remembered:

> The patients I had, I had an awful lot that were on Public Aid. . . . A lot of the public aid patients didn't have to pay anything. We got paid for two calls a month. My first office calls were $3 and for a house call it was something like $3. . . . they would only pay for two house calls a month. I had one lady who was on public aid, lived out at Holton Homes, and I used to have to go out and see her every week. She wanted to talk really. I knew her sons in high school, and really I would go out and give her a B12 shot once a week. One time I remember I tried to get her to let me send the nurse out for this shot. "No, Dr. Theobald, I've got to see you." So I would go out and sit there and talk with her for half hour or so, but I only got paid for two calls out of the four I would make.[98]

Medicare introduced both opportunities and challenges, particularly for rural practitioners. Russell Oyer remembered:

> Your people get older with you, so I was seeing . . . by the time I quit, a lot of the people were Medicare age — probably 60 percent. I had to stop doing OB and was doing some pediatrics, but I wasn't in the nursery any more for the last 10 or 15 years. So my pediatric population began dwindling. So I was . . . in a sense doing mostly geriatrics at the time I quit. That became a financial problem a little bit. Medicare never pays for what you — even though you follow the guidelines in charging, they never pay you. And cash flow began to be a little bit of a problem for me.[99]

According to Albert VanNess, in urban communities surgeons felt the greatest impact from the introduction of Medicare:

> When Medicare came through, the individual who had worked his life out here on the railroad or something. . . he

then decided he could get his hernia repaired. . . or take out the gallbladder. This is the first time they ever had the where-with-all to do anything like that. To see the family practitioner wasn't that expensive in the middle class anyway.[100]

During the years after World War II, the proportion of medical costs paid by both private and public insurance increased dramatically. Indeed, between 1960 and 1975, the share of health care expenses paid by third parties increased from 45 to 67 percent. Since virtually all insurance programs pay on the basis of fee-for-service, physicians had a significant incentive to increase both services and fees. With the involvement of third parties, which established rates of reimbursement according to usual, customary or prevailing rates, medical charges increased. According to one expert, "Fees began to soar when some young doctors, who had no record of charges, billed at unprecedented levels and were paid. When their older colleagues saw what was possible, they, too, raised their fees, and soon what was customary was higher than ever before." [101] Inflation of medical fees was also stimulated by increases in physicians' expenses for both medical training and malpractice insurance. These conditions affected young practitioners' earnings aspirations and their choice of practice location.

Dr. Theobald said of the newest generation of physicians, "They're good doctors, technically and all this. I hate to say it, but I think a lot of them are in it for the. . . money."[102] Russell Oyer amplified on this theme:

When I went into medicine, you hung up your shingle and you did it on your own. You were it! You were not going to be paid a salary. You were not going to have any benefits. You were a private and solo practice. Solo practice, of course, is going by the board now. Maybe that's good, I think. . . . Solo practice is probably a poor way to practice medicine from the point of view of stress and all that sort of thing. But I think that young physicians. . . are asking questions . . . these days. You know, "How much time will I have with my family? How much can I earn? How much vacation will I get? How many nights a week can I be off and away from the telephone?" I think these kinds of questions . . . didn't occur to us. Whether we were just naive. . . you expected that you were going to be . . . tied to your patients and that was your first loyalty and family or whatever came after that.[103]

Relationships With Patients

The physicians interviewed for this study experienced the height of patient dependence on physicians. Unlike their nineteenth-century forebears, they did not have to compete with a host of alternative practitioners or amateur healers. They agreed that patients tended to follow their advice. Indeed, Paul Theobald said, "Most of my patients were very good. If I told them to sit down and drop dead, they would sit down and drop dead."[104]

Interview respondents also agreed that the relationship between general practitioners and their patients was more satisfying than that between specialists and their patients. According to Harold Shinall, when he was a general practitioner, "I liked the people and the community, and I really liked the practice. I missed it a great deal after I got into my residency. It was not impersonal, yet you just saw patients that were referred to you and then you'd see some others. That was it."[105] Russell Oyer agreed, commenting about increasing specialization:

> I guess one of my chief concerns has been the human part of medicine, the personal part of medicine and how much does that mean to a patient? How much importance is it to a patient? Do we lose something if medicine becomes much more impersonal? I think some specialization, I think the way we manage patients with computers and numbers and all sorts of stuff. . . I think. . . as we learn more and as we do more, and as we fragment all the approaches to patients, somebody does this and somebody does that, I think the approach becomes less personal. The patient, I think, does get the impression, "Hey, I'm really just kind of a number here." I always used to have a strong feeling that the GP was the kind of person who needed to keep all that put together for the patient.[106]

From the physician's perspective, more damaging to the doctor-patient relationship than specialization has been the increase in malpractice litigation. Harold Shinall remembered, of his early days in practice:

> I was practicing several months in Gibson City without any insurance at all. Even at that time I wouldn't drive my car

around the block without insurance. There was a salesman from the Medical Protection Organization who drove through from Springfield one day and stopped in my office and asked if I would be interested in any insurance. I talked to him awhile and he sold me a policy. That was my first insurance plan.[107]

According to interview respondents, the trend toward malpractice litigation came to McLean County relatively late. Loren Boon recalled, "When I first started, why . . . no lawyer would take a malpractice suit here in McLean County. Patients had to go over to Peoria."[108]

Nonetheless, after the 1960s the threat of a malpractice suit hovered over physicians and affected the way they practiced medicine. Dr. Oyer said:

> I definitely worried about malpractice suits. I think that stimulated my effort to really make good notes in the office. . . . I became more concerned about being sure that any contact I had with a patient was recorded.
> *Interviewer*: So, not necessarily any particular event, just the whole climate.
> *Respondent*: Well, knowing colleagues for example who were sued, and being very dismayed when a colleague that I respected was sued for causes that I thought were totally unjust. Things that had no bearing on competency at all. That's one of the problems that you have. You know, an obstetrician getting sued for a very difficult breach delivery, for example. . . .[109]

Nurses also felt a change in the atmosphere of care after the increase of malpractice litigation. Alice Swift said, "I thought it was terrible. I felt like you couldn't be yourself. You couldn't be relaxed like you once were. . . . The thing that directed your care giving was whether or not there would be a law suit, not whether the patient was getting the kind of care he should get."[110]

From the physicians' perspective, the litigious atmosphere introduced an element of suspicion which had not been present before in the doctor-patient relationship. Dr. Livingston attributes this factor to the destructive activities of popular "health advisers":

> It is truly unfortunate. . . that the physician's greatest weapon against illness, whether organic or functional; namely, belief in the healing power possessed by the practi-

tioner, has been greatly diminished by the continuous encouragement of so-called popular "health advisers" for patients to challenge all decisions made for their treatment. Various medical mistakes are cited by these advisers to emphasize their position. Certainly errors do occur but these incidences are now magnified by publicity so that it would appear that most medical activities are fraught with improper care.[111]

Dr. Boon suggested that lawyers may have been partly to blame for stimulating malpractice suits, saying, "I think they probably got more trial lawyers here [in McLean County] and then they decided to keep some of the money themselves [rather] than refer them [the patients to lawyers in Peoria]."[112] It is also possible that rising health care costs forced families to sue in order to support devastating expenses for the long-term care of patients who failed to recover from either illness or medical treatment. Regardless of the reasons for increased malpractice litigation, this development has certainly contributed to the cost of health care by inflating the price of malpractice insurance.

Conclusions

The most significant change in twentieth-century health care has been an inflation of expectations regarding health and health care on the part of both medical practitioners and patients. In the years following the second World War, new medical discoveries and technical innovations were so frequent that they became commonplace. These developments touched the lives of all Americans — indeed, all humans coming into contact with Western medicine. In the heady days of the 1950s, 1960s and 1970s, there seemed to be no obstacle that could not be overcome — no age-old killer which could not be vanquished. The introduction of antibiotics in the mid-1940s appeared to herald the demise of infection as a threat to life; worldwide immunization campaigns reduced the incidence of polio in the 1950s and actually did away with smallpox in the 1970s. The development of transplant surgery meant that millions who would otherwise certainly have died have survived to enjoy productive lives; the introduction of bypass surgery in the 1950s improved the quality of life for countless sufferers from cardiovascular diseases.

It has been an age of miracles, and physicians have been the gatekeepers for these miracles. Sufferers have eagerly renounced traditional responsibility for health care decision-making, relying on the knowledge and power of doctors to solve their problems. No intervention has been too radical, no price too high, if the life of the premature baby, the desperately ill child, the beloved spouse or failing parent could be saved. Lay people have demanded the impossible of physicians; physicians have expected the impossible of themselves. Like spoiled children, sufferers assume that medicine can defeat illness, old age, even death, if only they can find the right doctor willing to perform the right magic trick.

These inflated expectations have created a health care delivery system which no one planned. The system has emphasized treatment of acute illness in institutional settings. It has made multi-million dollar businesses of health care institutions, provider networks and health insurance companies. Physicians and patients have become both the beneficiaries and the victims of this system. While enjoying unprecedented social status and financial rewards, physicians live in fear of being held accountable for impossible standards of performance. Specialization deprives them, as well as patients, of the full benefits of the unique relationship traditional between sufferers and healers. The cost-benefit impetus which drives the business of health care delivery imposes increasing restraints on physicians' ability to make therapeutic decisions based on individual patients' needs and limits patients' real choices about ways to manage birth, illness, and death.

This chapter has emphasized changes in professional medicine in McLean County during the twentieth century. However, it must end with the story unfinished. Perhaps the greatest changes are yet to come. As all concerned citizens recognize that professional health care has, in living memory, been transformed from a luxury to a necessity, we may be able imaginatively to muster the enormous resources of the community to face the challenges of the future. The old enemy still haunts us, appearing in many forms. AIDS, the newest contagious killer, mocks the hubris of daring to think that infectious disease is no longer dangerous. Cancer and cardiovascular diseases defy this century's Herculean efforts to vanquish them. However, a more significant challenge than combatting disease and death is that of overcoming the destructive facets of human nature. We must muster both collective and individual will power to defeat the sloth, self indulgence, and venality generating our self-inflicted wounds. Obesity, substance abuse, teenage pregnancy, and many cancers can be prevented. So can the barriers to accessing high quality health care, which include poverty, ignorance, and greed.

In Living Memory: The Experience of Health, Illness and Medical Care in McLean County

When I was sick and lay abed,
I had two pillows at my head,
And all my toys beside me lay
To keep me happy all the day.

And sometimes for an hour or so
I watched my leaden soldiers go,
With different uniforms and drills
Among the bedclothes, through the hills;

And sometimes sent my ships in fleets
All up and down among the sheets;
Or brought my trees and houses out,
And planted cities all about.

I was the giant great and still
That sits upon the pillow-hill
And sees before him, dale and plain,
The pleasant Land of Counterpane.

Robert Louis Stevenson,
"The Pleasant Land of Counterpane"
(first published in 1885)

In living memory, the experience of suffering and healing has changed dramatically. The diseases people most feared and those they died of were very different at the beginning than they are at the end of this century. The power of professional medicine to alter the course of disease and delay death grew beyond the wildest fantasies of nineteenth-century healers and sufferers. During the brief span of one or two generations, management of birth, illness, and death moved from homes to medical institutions, and from the realm of family members to that of experts. This chapter explores these changes from the perspective of McLean County residents who lived through them.

It depends on oral history interviews conducted with 39 people born between 1894 and 1966.[1] Nearly three-quarters of respondents are female; just over one-quarter are African American. Twenty-two interviewees have spent most of their lives in Bloomington-Normal; 15 have lived mainly in rural communities.

Table 1
Oral history respondents: date of birth and gender

Date of birth	Males	Females
1890-1900	0	3
1901-1910	2	4
1911-1920	5	10
1920-1930	3	8
1931-1940	0	2
1941-1950	0	1
1951-1960	0	0
1961-1970	0	1
Total	10	29

Respondents were selected within three primary occupational categories to obtain information about attitudes toward and experience of ill-health and medical care from both professional and lay points of view. Eight nurses, six physicians, and one dentist were interviewed, as were 24 lay people whose occupations include domestic service, teaching, factory work, journalism, farming, insurance, medical records management, and housewifery. Since health care practitioners talked about their own experiences of ill-health and childbearing in addition to their professional activities, their memories are discussed along with those of lay people.

Educational attainment of respondents ranged from three years of high school to professional graduate degrees. Although no information about interviewees' income was elicited, interviews reveal that while many respondents experienced poverty as children and young adults, most of them currently enjoy moderate or high incomes and comparatively comfortable lifestyles.

The oral history respondents come from a range of socioeconomic, ethnic, racial and religious backgrounds. They represent both rural and urban experience. Their memories cover a period of almost a century. The preponderance of females among interviewees is useful because of women's traditional role as decision-makers regarding matters of health in most households. Although most respondents have lived in McLean County all their lives, it may be argued that their experience is typical of residents of small cities and rural communities throughout the American mid-

midwest. As the development of the County's health care delivery system conformed, generally speaking, to the national model, changes in respondents' beliefs, behavior and experience regarding health, illness, birth, and medical care also illustrate broad cultural trends.

Fear, Self-Defense, and Resignation: Infections and People

During the first half of the twentieth century, the phrase "childhood diseases" did not suggest the mild discomfort and interrupted schedules met with relative equanimity by today's parents. Instead, these ailments were savage monsters, killing and maiming indiscriminately, and leaving a legacy of terror and grief in their wake. Although immunization against smallpox and diphtheria was possible, outbreaks of these and other contagious diseases were publicly dealt with as short-term crises; there were no concerted efforts to immunize children. Born in 1914, Caribel Washington remembered, "When I was in the eighth grade . . . , there was quite an epidemic of smallpox. Our teacher had it, so then everybody had to be vaccinated."[2] Indeed, because vaccines and immunization procedures were not well refined, people feared them. Grace Allman, born in 1896, remembered being vaccinated against smallpox as a teenager:

> Everybody had to get vaccinated for smallpox. That was a bad experience for me too because when I got vaccinated, my arm swelled up and it was that big.
> *Interviewer*: What happened? Do you know why it did that?
> *Respondent*: It was just sore. I was teaching, and to go to school I carried my arm, I fastened my thumb in my belt so that I had no weight on this.[3]

Perhaps, in part, because of the fear of the immunization process, despite the availability of smallpox vaccine and diphtheria antitoxin at the time, there were 140 reported cases of smallpox in Bloomington in 1925 and 89 cases of diphtheria in 1921.[4]

Other contagious diseases could not as easily be prevented. Very infectious and always present, measles was epidemic in some years; in 1925, 771 cases were reported in Bloomington. Whooping cough and scarlet fever were also endemic, more virulent in some years than in others. New to Illinois in 1917, poliomyelitis, also referred to as infantile paralysis, began to visit McLean County on a regular basis; 22 cases were reported to the State Health Department in 1927, 20 cases in 1931.[5]   Mainly striking otherwise healthy children, and crippling those it did not kill, polio was feared out of all proportion to its incidence.

In addition to infections which mainly threatened children, there were contagious diseases which were less discriminating. Although the number of cases declined steadily in the early twentieth century, tuberculosis remained a constant threat. Pneumonia also continued to claim lives, particularly as a complication of other diseases. For example, during the influenza epidemic of 1918, in addition to 83 deaths in Bloomington from flu, 57 people — more than twice the number reported the following year — died of pneumonia. Typhoid was also a regular visitor to the County, as were the sexually transmitted diseases syphilis and gonorrhea.[6]

With the exception of tuberculosis sufferers cared for at the Fairview Sanitarium, victims of the 1918 influenza epidemic nursed in the temporary hospital set up in the clubhouse at Bloomington Country Club, and polio patients hospitalized, first at St. Francis Hospital in Peoria, later at St. Joseph's Hospital in Bloomington, sufferers from infectious diseases were looked after at home.[7] Visited by physicians, nursed by mothers, other female relatives or servants, the sick either recovered or died in their own beds. Diphtheria could be treated with antitoxin; beginning in the 1930s, pneumonia could sometimes be cured by sulfa drugs. Paul Ehrlich's formulation of Salvarsan in 1911 made syphilis curable.[8] Otherwise, no effective treatments were available for most infections. Sufferers were comforted and watched. The healthy were protected from contagion by strictly observed quarantine of the ill and personal hygiene procedures intended to limit the spread of germs increasingly became part of the general education of children.

A booklet, *Home Care of Communicable Diseases*, published in 1942 by the John Hancock Mutual Life Insurance Company, provides a revealing glimpse of contemporary management of infectious illnesses before the introduction of antibiotics and well coordinated and utilized immunization campaigns. Directed at mothers of young children, this publication provided information in simple language about symptoms of major childhood diseases, the ways infections were spread, and development of immunity to some diseases. It debunked outdated ideas about infection:

People, not things, usually spread communicable diseases. Saliva is the chief agent which carries the infection. Until recent times there were differences of opinion about the transmission of disease. Our forefathers thought the infectious agent was the night air itself. Sewer gases were wrongly accused of spreading diseases. Peeling skin from recovered cases was mistakenly thought to be dangerous.[9]

The booklet indicates how quickly "modern" ideas can become outdated, maintaining, for example, that German Measles (or rubella) has no common complications. Ironically, it was in 1941 that the Australian, Norman McAlister Gregg, first identified a connection between rubella occurring during pregnancy and birth defects.[10]

The booklet recommends that sufferers from infectious diseases be put to bed in a room by themselves, partly to speed recovery and partly to protect other members of the household. Patients were to be completely isolated until all danger of infection had passed; thus, they were to use a bedpan rather than the bathroom and to eat all their meals in bed. The booklet stresses the importance of keeping babies and preschoolers away from the patient, because "communicable diseases go especially hard for youngsters between the ages of six months and three or four years. Most deaths from these diseases occur among babies and toddlers."[11] Regardless of the disease, the nurse was instructed to:

Wear a large apron while caring for the patient and leave the apron always in the sickroom;
Wash hands thoroughly after caring for the patient;
Turn away from the patient when he coughs or sneezes and keep own hands away from mouth.

Additional special precautions were necessary in nursing people suffering from diphtheria, polio, scarlet fever and smallpox:

All articles used by the patient must be kept in the sick room or until they can be burned, boiled, soaked in disinfectant solution, or aired. Soiled linen should be washed in soap and hot water apart from the family wash and unnecessary handling avoided.
Dishes should be boiled for fifteen minutes before being washed with the household dishes. Partly eaten scraps of food should be burned.

Special procedures were followed for disposal of the excrement of sufferers from ailments, such as polio and typhoid, which were transmitted by fecal matter. After the patient had recovered, the sickroom was to be thoroughly cleaned and aired. In addition, "All articles such as mattress, blankets, or books should be put in the sun for at least six hours. Articles badly soiled, of course, should be cleaned or destroyed if they cannot be cleaned."[12] This booklet described an ideal. In fact, what oral history respondents remembered was quarantining; they also remember the outcomes of bouts with contagious diseases.

Regardless of precautions taken, these ailments continued to kill. Ruth Carpenter, born in 1909, remembered a diphtheria epidemic which visited her rural community when she was a child:

> We had a neighbor down the road. . . and the family got diphtheria and one of the little girls died, and that [household] was quarantined. And when she died they brought the body outside, . . . they brought it from the funeral home and . . . set it out in the front yard.
> *Interviewer*: Did people come, and . . . ?
> *Respondent*: Yeah, they did. Oh, everybody was so kind and they brought stuff. Of course they didn't go in the house. . . . But I can remember the quarantine signs. . . .
> *Interviewer*: And who put them up?
> *Respondent*: The doctor, I guess the doctor that took care of 'em and reported it. As far as I know it was when the doctor reported it then they hung the sign on. And they treated you like you had the plague. . . . Oh, yes. They was scared to death of you.[13]

Reginald Whitaker, born in 1925, remembered that his mother had been married as a young woman to a man named John Duff who died of typhoid:

> He died, I think, he died in 1907. My mother was carrying John; he never saw his father. She was seven months pregnant, or something like that. He died. . . John was born in 1907. . . .
> *Interviewer*: He must have been quite a young man, Mr. Duff.
> *Respondent*: 21. . . . They had a typhoid fever epidemic, you understand, going through the Twin Cities at that time.[14]

Grace Allman, born in 1896, said that her husband's family was decimated by influenza. "His mother and a sister died with the flu. My husband was so ill they thought he was going to die. They were buried the same day, his sister and his mother."[15]

Martha Ferguson, born in 1916, remembered the general fear of epidemic diseases:

> Scarlet fever was terrifying, you know. Anything like that was really pretty dangerous. They didn't really have any good cures for anything.
> *Interviewer*: How did your family and the community deal with these problems?
> *Respondent*: Well, we were just taken care of at home. They quarantined. . . for a lot of things in those days. Scarlet fever was always quarantined. I think chicken pox was. I think whooping cough was. . . . Well, we were scared of scarlet fever; yeah, you could get pretty ill from that and people did die.[16]

Even when contagious diseases did not kill, they created a major disruption in people's lives. Marie Bostic, born in 1897, taught in a one-room school as a young woman and caught scarlet fever from one of her students:

> They sent that kid to school that morning with a terrible sore throat. He was just a little boy and was just a-crying. I had him on my lap most of the day. I'd rather hold him as to have him cry. That was on Friday. Sunday morning I had scarlet fever. I caught it from him. We were quarantined five weeks. There was no school for six weeks.[17]

Mary Finfgeld remembered being quarantined with influenza at about age 12 during the 1918 epidemic:

> [I was in] that bedroom in the house and nobody came in there, and I mean *nobody* came in there, excepting my mother to look after me and bring me my meals. Nobody even stuck their head in the door. It was . . . well, I haven't ever seen anything like it since, because people, they were just dropping dead like flies.[18]

As remains the case today, little could be done for flu sufferers;

aspirin and bedrest were the only treatments used.

Tuberculosis was endemic rather than epidemic. Although mortality from the disease declined during the early twentieth century due to improved living standards and measures taken to isolate the sick from the well, it remained a significant threat. Ferne Hensley, born in 1894, talked about tuberculosis in her family. Her aunt had died of the disease at the age of 14:

> She was a tiny little girl. She died of what they called consumption — TB, you know. . . . Well, I guess it sort of just consumed them. One of my father's — next to the oldest brother — he also died with it. A number of people. Of course, there were no sanitariums or anything like that. They just — you had it and that was it. You didn't get well from it then.[19]

Younger respondents remembered friends and relatives receiving treatment for tuberculosis at the Fairview Sanitarium. Reginald Whitaker remembered friends of his sister — a brother and sister from Bloomington — who suffered from TB:

> They were both out there at McLean County Tuberculosis Center. Her brother got along real well, came out, and I guess didn't do what he was supposed to and he died. Got very infected. Didn't follow the doctor's orders, as far as I can remember. She's still living. This would have been back in the '30s, the middle '30s. She stayed out there in that sanitarium — she had to learn to walk all over again. *Interviewer*: Because she'd been in bed so long? *Respondent*: Yeah. Been in bed two or three years. But she finally got out. I don't know how long she was there. . . . I think back then they would collapse a lung and let that rest. . . . They collapsed the one and waited until it healed. Then they put it back in action and collapsed the other. I think that's what took so long. She had to learn to walk all over again.[20]

Although surgical treatments were developed for tuberculosis in the 1920s, there was no reliable drug therapy until the late 1940s when streptomycin was introduced.[21]

In addition to diseases such as tuberculosis, which still threaten residents of McLean County, oral history respondents remember suffering from illnesses which, due to public health measures or the introduction of effective treatments, have virtually disappeared. Mary Finfgeld, born in 1906, suffered from undulant fever, also called brucellosis, in the early 1940s. She recalled:

> You get it from cow's milk. I had always been taught
> that you never use anything but pasteurized milk, but
> when we moved here a man out in the country had dairy
> cows and . . . left a quart of milk on our back porch. So I
> continued to take some milk from him, but I bought pas-
> teurized milk for the children. . . . It [the brucellosis] was
> traced to his herd, one cow. . . .
> *Interviewer*: You said you had a fever of 105?
> *Respondent*: At one time when it spiked highest. They put
> me in the hospital then. I went to bed on December 7,
> 1941, Pearl Harbor Day, and I got out at Easter time. And
> you carry that in your system all your life. So I've never
> been able to give blood. But I haven't had any more trouble
> with it. They had no medication for it at that time. Doc
> Ryder consulted with Mayo's and they had nothing. Within
> two years they had a vaccine. You got one shot in your hip
> and one in your arm. . . . There were a few cases of that
> around in the area and one man had died from it, but I did-
> n't know that at the time. But I guess I had people plenty
> worried — though I never thought I was that sick.[22]

Undulant fever was a debilitating disease which lasted a long time. Mrs. Rittenhouse contracted it in the late 1940s as a child:

> I was probably pretty healthy until I was six, seven or eight
> — somewhere in there. My father milked cows and at that
> time you did not pasteurize the milk, and I got undulant
> fever, which is called milk fever. I was sick for probably a
> year or two. And I remember going down to Mennonite
> Hospital in Bloomington and being checked and things.
> And I remember them moving my bed from upstairs down
> stairs in the living room, because I had to be in bed all the
> time. You know, you don't remember how long it took. I
> don't remember how long I was sick, but I know that I
> spent several months being sick like that and it took a long
> time to get strength back and everything. And I think at
> the time my father came down with it too. So we were both
> not well during that time.[23]

Brucellosis largely disappeared as pasteurization became universal among dairy farmers and the general public stopped drinking untreated milk.

The incidence of other life-threatening and debilitating diseases diminished with the introduction of antibiotics. Caribel Washington remembered having rheumatic fever in 1939:

> I was quite ill. I was on crutches and I limped, and I had a cane, and all of these kind of things. It was from an infected throat. I never had any heart problems because it moved all over my body.... I think that's why I have such a heavy tolerance for pain. I used to sit for a half hour just making up my mind to get up. It was excruciating....
> *Interviewer*: What was really done for you?
> *Respondent*: The biggest thing I took was salicylate acid.... I used to go out to — when St. Joseph was still up here, I'd go and they would put me in a cabinet and close it clear up to my neck up here, and then turn on these electric lights and then stand there and feed me ice water so I would sweat.
> *Interviewer*: You were lying down?
> *Respondent*: No. There was a chair. And you'd just go in that cabinet and they'd just close the whole thing up and your head was out. It would close up to your neck and you were just in a cabinet. When they did that they would take me downstairs and have pans of wet salt. They'd use scrub brushes to rub that salt into my skin because they said the pores were full of this poison. Then they would — and this one I couldn't take — they'd put me in a bathtub and put electrodes in the tub, you know, but that made me sick at the stomach, so I couldn't take that at the time.... But this cabinet bit, oh dear.
> *Interviewer*: And there were lights, you said, so it was hot?
> *Respondent*: Right. There was all different types of watts of lights that were inside. When I would get in there and they would close it up and then they would turn that on. Then heat would get in there.... I always felt better after that... because they did it until I would sweat a certain amount. The more I sweated, the more that would leave my system.[24]

A disease caused by streptococci bacteria, rheumatic fever was both treated and effectively prevented by the use of antibiotics beginning in the 1940s.

According to Dr. Harold Shinall, who worked as a general practitioner in Gibson City during the 1930s, the majority of the patients he attended suffered from infections.[25] Judging from oral evidence, his experience was typical. Lay people most frequently recalled consulting physicians for acute infectious illnesses. For example, Richard Finfgeld, born in 1906, remembered his brother Ray suffering from a serious upper respiratory infection as a young man:

> They didn't think he was going to live. Dr. Hammers was his doctor. He was coming to our house to see and take care of him [Ray]. As I remember it, he had pneumonia or something. He had a high temperature. They put a plaster on his chest. . . . This wasn't a mustard plaster. This was something milder. It was supposed to be something good. They were so concerned they called in Dr. Scott. The two doctors came to our house and had a consultation. Dr. Scott suggested or ordered that they change to put on a mustard plaster. . . . That was the second plaster. . . . He was really afflicted. They didn't think he was going to live, but he recovered. . . . But nobody ever went to the hospital. When people died, they died in their homes.[26]

As important as the doctor's advice was the support of friends and relatives during times of serious illness. Lavada Hunter, born in 1913, remembered:

> What I can remember about death was, the first time I was 10 years of age. My father died then. . . . In 1923 he had the influenza. He was at home, and the family doctor would come and attend him before death came. During those days, people used to sit up with the sick. They would come and help my mother with him, you know, in many many ways. They helped cook, wash, and iron. I was ten years old, and I counted twenty people at our home when my father was so very ill. Then was when my mother found out that she thought that he was dying. He was in a delirious state. Then he died; he finally died at home.[27]

This kind of lay community support was quite traditional, declining only when hospitalization of women in childbirth, the very sick, and the dying became usual.

Indeed, in the early years of the century, some families managed most illnesses on their own, without consulting physicians. Ruth Carpenter said, "My father was allergic to doctors, I think. . . . He didn't believe in going to the doctor. . . . He just said they didn't have any good common sense."[28] Her family relied extensively on home remedies, calling the doctor only as a last resort.

Self-Dosing: Home Remedies and Patent Medicines

Whether or not their families consulted physicians, most respondents born before about 1940 remembered using home remedies. The memory of herbal remedies is particularly strong among African American respondents, perhaps because of a sturdy cultural tradition, perhaps because of the difficulties African Americans have encountered until comparatively recently in obtaining professional medical care. Lucinda Brent Posey, born in 1914, remembered:

> Every Fall, I had to go with Grandma . . . to get her roots for bitters. A bottle and a blue granite kettle were kept on the top shelf of the pantry for this. Hickory bark from the tree, dandelion roots, plantain roots, and I don't know what other kind of roots went into the bitters. Grandma spent the next day scraping and cleaning her roots. They were put in the blue granite kettle with water and simmered all day; strained through a cheese cloth. Eventually, the brown liquid went into the tall bottle. Mother was told to bring home one-half pint of whiskey. It was poured into the bottle. If your toe hurt, you got a teaspoonful; if your head hurt, you got a teaspoonful; the same for a stomachache. I learned *never* to complain; the pain was not nearly so bad as taking the bitters.[29]

Mrs. Caribel Washington, also African American and born in 1914, recalled:

> My dad's mother was a kind of a herb doctor. They could go out in the yard and find several leaves that were good for sores, and good for bathing the feet or poulticing different places and that sort of thing. . . . They believed in ginseng weed and pope berries. When pope berries were ripe, they would make a kind of tonic out of that.[30]

White respondents also remembered herbal remedies. Grace Allman, born in 1896, recalled her mother's recipe for cough syrup:

> Well, honey and horehound. I don't know what else was in it. She'd make it and a great big bottle would always sit up in the cupboard. If we had a cough or a cold we had the cough medicine ready.... Now, my husband's mother used to use whiskey in medicine that she made, but my mother didn't believe in that.[31]

Ralph Spencer, born in 1914, remembered his mother using tonics based on humoral ideas of disease prevention:

> My mother always had a remedy for whatever it was. In the spring of the year she had a blood thinner that she gave you, and things like that.
> *Interviewer*: Can you describe any of those?
> *Respondent*: Well . . . , for blood thinner we used sassafras tea and stuff like that. The mint is strong and that would thin your blood.[32]

Herbs were used externally as well as internally. Both Lucinda Brent Posey and Caribel Washington remembered wearing asafetida bags around their necks as children to ward off illness. Washington said, "I guess everybody wore them. I know we always had them."[33]

Remedies were also made of common kitchen ingredients and household substances. Many people born before 1920 , white and black, remember a cough syrup described by Ruth Carpenter:

> [My stepmother] had an old teacup. It was still useable and she put a big onion in there and maybe sectioned it off and covered it with sugar and then set it on the back of the cookstove and made it simmer. And it made a good cough syrup.[34]

Onions were also used in poultices for congested chests and sore throats. Lucinda Brent Posey remembered the onion being "heated, put into a piece of cotton sheeting, and put on your chest when you had a chest cold."[35] Ruth Carpenter recalled applying poultices made of bread and milk to "draw" local infections.[36] Martha Ferguson, born in 1916, remembered, "For the nail in my foot they used a home remedy which consisted of burning wool in a shovel and putting my foot over the smoke."[37]

Lucinda Brent Posey recalled another poultice composed of an easily accessible substance:

> The final remedy of *all* remedies was when I had the flu in 1918. A cow manure poultice was made and put on my chest. Mother went somewhere with an old kettle and got the cow manure. Grandma heated it, put it into white sheeting, and (despite my screams and hollers) put the *hot* stinky poultice on my chest. It was covered with a piece of flannel to hold in the heat. Despite all of that, I was better in the morning and the cough loosened up.[38]

Caribel Washington remembered her family using home remedies for colds:

> We always had coal oil glycerin that we took for a bad cold. . . . I guess they don't call it coal oil these days, do they? What do they call it? Kerosene! When we were children they called it coal oil, but it was kerosene and glycerin. They would mix some portion of that up in a big bottle and then if you had a cold, . . . shake that bottle up and give you some of that. They believed in goose grease. They thought goose grease had some curative powers to it.[39]

Many respondents remembered rubbing turpentine on injuries. According to Ruth Carpenter:

> We had a bottle in the house for the humans and another for the horses out in the barn.
> *Interviewer*: What would you do with it? You'd just rub it on the injured part?
> *Respondent*: Well, yeah, or pour it. If it was an open wound you just poured it on. It made it burn like crazy.[40]

Respondents also remembered home cures for croup. Ruth Carpenter's stepmother would soak a towel in cold water, "wrap it around my neck and it [croup] would soon disappear."[41] Harking back to the sympathetic magic of the past, Ethel Cherry, born in 1911, remembered, "My brother used to have croup all the time and my mother put a silk thread around his neck to keep him from having croup. And it worked!"[42]

206

In addition to remedies made at home, many people took patent medicines, purchased over the counter. Margaret Esposito, born in 1923, recalled that her father had the reputation within his own family for being something of a hypochondriac:

> I can remember him having a propensity for some kinds of over-the-counter drugs. I don't remember now what they were.
> *Interviewer*: Do you remember him regularly taking tonics or laxatives, say?
> *Respondent*: Yes. . . . I can't say what they were or anything. I think the most ridiculous thing that happened that I can remember rather distinctly . . . . I was then grown and he was having an upset stomach and he went to the cabinet and got out a bottle of pink fluid and thought it Pepto Bismol and it was . . .Caladryl. . . . He took a swig of that and just was shocked.[43]

Her father also regularly spent his summer vacations at a spa in Missouri, "taking the baths. . . . And drinking the water and that sort of thing," in an effort to improve his health.

Ruth Carpenter, born in 1909, remembered her family purchasing patent remedies from traveling salesmen:

> In those days, we had Raleigh men and McNess men and, what was the other one. . . ? They . . . would come traveling through the countryside with their . . . big bag. . . . And they had, like, mentholatum salve and . . . carbolic salve and then he had just a little of everything. Oh, it was wonderful for that man to come.[44]

She remembered her father taking a laxative called a "Hinkle pill," saying, "He thought it would cure anything." She said that a lot of older people prevented and cured illness by doing "what they called purging themselves. . . . That was a regular practice."[45]

Marie Bostic, born in 1897, recalled buying a tonic from a traveling peddler, saying, "We'd go to the show they had."[46] A number of respondents remember being given castor oil or cod liver oil as children to ward off illness.

In the days before the introduction of antibiotics, home or patent remedies were often the only treatments available, regardless of the seriousness of the patient's illness. Caribel Washington remembered her mother suffering from pneumonia:

She was a big beautiful woman, but she got pneumonia and those were . . . the days when you didn't send people to the hospitals. We were so afraid she was going to die. . . . We would take 1/2 gallon fruit jars and put big gobs of Vicks salve in and pour boiling water over it, you know, to set up the vapor in the room for her. In those days, they put a flannel jacket on a person, and you didn't take that off, unless for bathing or something. We just always felt that those were the things as much as anything else that helped our mother. I don't recall the medicine that she took. She must have taken some. I can just remember how religiously we would boil that water and just keep it hot to help her.[47]

Mrs. Washington also recalled dosing her own son with patent remedies used when she was a child. "You see, as children, we believed a lot in quinine. . . . And Castor oil was always in our house. I can't ever recall an aspirin, but back in those days it was quinine. We did a lot with it. So, whatever we gave him [for scarlet fever], he got better."[48]

Family members and friends shared the responsibility for health care decisions with any medical practitioners they consulted. They also provided the lion's share of patient care. Dr. Loren Boon, who began practicing medicine in Danvers in 1947, remembered that the frail elderly and terminally ill had been looked after at home in the early years of his practice:

Of course, when I very first started there were a lot of families that still had people at home there, and there was always a maiden aunt or somebody at home to help take care of them . . . . And then after awhile everybody had to work that was at home . . . .[49]

Boon focused on social and economic changes affecting availability of home care. However, equally significant was the shift from customary dependence on home care and comforts in times of illness to reliance on medical professionals and high-tech institutional resources to manage all major challenges to health.

Patients and Doctors

Even in an era when home care was the rule, families developed long-standing relationships with local doctors. Richard Finfgeld, who lived in Lexington during the 1910s and 1920s, remembered that, although people virtually never went to hospitals, they did consult the four doctors then serving the community of approximately 1,500:

> The doctors . . . had their offices there in town and they made house calls. Not only house calls in Lexington but they had all the rural territory. My older brother Cliff, he was chauffeur for Dr. Hammers and they had a Hudson car. He was responsible for keeping that car ready to go and he would drive that doctor all over the country and that was a problem, because there were no paved roads and there were no gravel roads to speak of. There might have been a little gravel around, but most of them were just mud roads. And he had a problem to get to see some of these people.[50]

Most of the doctors mentioned by respondents were general practitioners who delivered babies, set bones, did minor surgery and dealt with a variety of internal ailments. They were not expected to be able to solve all health problems, but rather to use their comparatively limited resources to combat disease to the best of their abilities. The doctor-patient relationship was built on trust which, in many cases, withstood even the implication that something was wrong about the doctor's methods. For example, Grace Allman consulted a physician in the village of Stanford whose office was, by some people, considered rather unsanitary. "In fact, the health department came up and inspected his office at one time and suggested that he change things." When she had a growth on her leg, her adult niece, "a physical education teacher . . . [who] thought she knew quite a few of the rules" advised her against having this doctor remove it because, "I might get . . . blood poisoning or something, you know. I ought to go some place else. I did have enough faith in Dr. Cavins so I didn't think that would happen."[51] She went ahead with the surgery, which was performed in Dr. Cavins' office.

To some extent, Grace Allman's trust was based on her personal relationship with the doctor and his wife. When she was in her early teens, Dr. and Mrs. Cavins were newlyweds:

> His wife was from Baltimore and that was horse and buggy days of course. When he had to make a call, she was kind of timid and didn't like to stay by herself, so he would come down and get me, and I would go up and sit with her. If he didn't get home very early, they invited me to stay for supper. I was always real happy to eat supper with them.[52]

Personal relationships also sometimes affected a doctor's failure to attract a substantial clientele. Richard Finfgeld said:

> I'll tell you about the medical situation. We had two MDs in Lexington; one was Dr. Hammers and one was Dr. Scott. A little later Dr. Scott's son graduated and was an MD and he came there and they practiced together and we had three at one time. That was three men and we had one woman. Her name was Dr. Bull. . . .
> *Interviewer*: Did this woman have her own practice?
> *Respondent*: In her home. The other two had offices downtown.
> *Interviewer*: Do you know how she was educated?
> *Respondent*: No. I don't know anything about her. I knew who she was and where she lived, but I didn't know anything about her. The others were licensed MDs.
> *Interviewer*: Do you suppose she was licensed also?
> *Respondent*: I think she must have been.
> *Interviewer*: She wasn't considered a quack?
> *Respondent*: No, I don't think so, but I don't think she was very popular.[53]

According to the McLean County Medical Society's *Biographical History,* Dr. E. Martha Bull was born in 1867 in Lexington and graduated from Northwestern University Woman's College in 1895. "She was in active practice until 1928 in Lexington, when because of serious illness was able to resume practice only in a modest way."[54] Her lack of popularity may have been due to her isolation from the close community of male practitioners, who had offices in town and consulted with each other on difficult cases. It is also possible that her gender made her comparatively less acceptable to prospective patients:

> *Interviewer*: Why probably was the female physician not well accepted?
> *Respondent*: I think maybe they didn't regard her as an authority. I don't really know what the adults thought about it. I knew she was just kind of off on the side there and didn't seem to be in the loop. But why they would come to that conclusion, I wouldn't know.
> *Interviewer*: Were there specific types of patients that might go to her?
> *Respondent*: Certain kinds of people, maybe, rather than

certain kinds of patients. People that maybe were not in the ordinary flow of the community. People who would be a little odd or something. . . . I don't know. But she just didn't have a wide practice that I knew of.[55]

Generally speaking, respondents who grew up in rural areas were treated by a physician who was located nearby. This proximity was advantageous both to physicians, who routinely made house calls, and to patients who had to either wait for a doctor's visit or travel to the office. As Ethel Cherry, born in 1911, said, "You didn't go a hundred miles to see a doctor. You just went to the doctor that was close to you." In her case, a seven-mile distance was involved.[56] Respondents living in Bloomington-Normal also remembered seeing local physicians. Reginald Whitaker, born in 1925, grew up in Normal. When asked if people traveled to Bloomington to see the doctor, he answered:

> No. All the doctors were doctors here. . . . Dr. Doud was here, Dr. Penniman. . . . They had doctors in Bloomington. I guess some people would go to Bloomington. . . . Dr. Doud was on North Street. Up over, you know, where the ice cream store is down there? Used to be Velvet Freeze, they called it. . . . He was upstairs there. Dr. McCormick, he was upstairs there too.[57]

Older respondents remembered calling the doctor more rarely than younger interviewees. Martha Ferguson, born in 1916, said that her family physician came to her house very seldom:

> *Interviewer*: But he did come occasionally?
> *Respondent*: He came for my sister's birth — my youngest sister's. And he came when we had scarlet fever. He even came when I had pneumonia, but those were so far apart.[58]

Nonetheless, most had a good deal of faith in doctors. Reginald Whitaker said, "My parents . . . didn't have a lot of foolish . . . ideas. If there was sickness and it didn't go away in a reasonable time, we'd have to get the doctor."[59] They also tended to take physicians' advice when it was given. Grace Allman explained, "If I go to the doctor and pay him money, I want to do what he says or else I wouldn't waste my money."[60]

In most families, mothers made the decision about whether

or not to call the doctor. According to Ralph Spencer, born in 1914:

> Well, my mother always said, "I think it's time," to my dad, "that you take Ralph or . . . Orville to see the doctor."
> *Interviewer*: Your dad never made that decision?"
> *Respondent*: Oh, no. He did whatever she told him to do in regards to something like that — oh yeah. He was the one that took you; she didn't.[61]

Since adult women also did most of the informal diagnosing and nursing within the home, they tended to have more experience and knowledge about illness than men.

Other female relatives also became involved in medical decision making. On a number of occasions, Reginald Whitaker's older sister, who lived in Chicago, took him to a doctor when he visited her as a child. "Now, my sister, Fay, had taken me to doctors downtown [in Chicago] when I was much smaller. She was always taking me to the doctor." He and another sister, Josephine, developed a rare eye condition which blinded both of them as mature adults. He recalled:

> You don't find many sisters that will do these things for you like she did. Like I said, she was like a second mother to me.
> *Interviewer*: Well, it sounds like she had a very strong personality.
> *Respondent*: Oh she did! Very strong willed. . . . She would take me and Josephine, whichever one of us would be up there, to a doctor. She took very good care of herself. Whenever she would go to a doctor's for herself, she would talk about Josephine and I.[62]

Because of a number of chronic health conditions, Mr. Whitaker had more experience with medical specialists than was common for people of his generation. As a child, he suffered severely from a skin condition, variously diagnosed as eczema and psoriasis. His older sister, who lived in Chicago, mentioned this problem to her doctor, a general practitioner, who "said he would take me to a friend of his, Dr. Thatcher was his name, a skin specialist. . . . He came by my sister's apartment on Sunday morning and picked me up and took me over to Dr. Thatcher's."[63] The specialist prescribed a salve which gave him temporary relief; however, the prescription did not work the next time the condition recurred.

212

As children, Reginald Whitaker and his sister Josephine also began to experience symptoms of the rare eye condition which eventually blinded them:

> *Interviewer*: When did you find out about that?
> *Respondent*: My mother noticed. She'd tell us to pick up something off the floor at night, and we'd be feeling around for it and she knew something was wrong. So we were taken to an optometrist . . . no, an eye doctor. . . .
> *Interviewer*: A specialist, an opthalmologist?
> *Respondent*: Yeah. They said, "Oh, it's night blindness." We were fine in the daylight or with lights on. I even used to drive at night. So we went for years thinking we had night blindness. . . .

In 1948, at age 23, Reginald was examined at the Illinois Eye and Ear Infirmary in Chicago:

> I was going up there once a month or maybe twice a month, [for] about three months for different examinations. Doctors were coming in from around the state and other states; for cases like mine they would have them come in and those doctors would examine us. . . . But nobody ever came up with what the problem is. . . . My sister, Fay, had heard about . . . a doctor who had set up practice there in Chicago and that he was very good. She was gonna have her eyes tested for new glasses. She went to him and told him about Josephine and I. He said, "I sure would like to see them when they're in the city again." So we were up there one Saturday and she called him and said we were there. . . . He was in his office on Saturdays, and then you could go at 7:00 on Saturday evening and he was there until 9:00. . . . So we went out there to his office and he examined us. Then he said, "You don't have night blindness." Boy, that sure felt good. "But! We call this retinitis pigmatosa and we don't know what to do for it. . . ." Then he wanted to know our family history. He said it's inherited, it's somewhere back in your family. . . . So he worked with us and tried different things. He would give us some kind of serum that they get from hogs. He was trying to . . . do a little experimental chemistry on Josephine. I think it did help her. She'd take about a shot a week, an injection. She spent the summer up there so she could go

get some medicine orally.... I didn't go through it. I was working and all.... Dr. James Richardson was his name. I understand he was one of the finest opthalmologists...! He was more of a scientist than really a doctor. He didn't have any bedside manner. But he was really a wonderful eye doctor....[64]

Mr. Whitaker's experience indicates the extent to which medical specialists were increasingly accessible in the mid-twentieth century, although it is significant that he consulted specialists located in Chicago. According to Dr. Albert VanNess, who began practicing as an internist in Bloomington in 1957, in those days, "Specialists didn't go to a town [with a population of] less than one million. I say that with tongue in cheek, but there weren't any specialists in Bloomington on the medical side. They were all generalists."[65] Reginald Whitaker's experience also illustrates the escalating belief that doctors could diagnose and find a cure for almost any condition. With enormous patience, he and his sister devoted a great deal of time and scarce financial resources to explore the medical options for dealing with their failing vision — a problem which in earlier times would probably have been met with a greater degree of fatalism and resignation.

Paying the Doctor

Although many of the oral history respondents remember having grown up in households where there was very little money, paying the doctor was not mentioned as a major problem. In the first half of the twentieth century, doctor bills were very low. Caribel Washington said:

> We ran across a receipt.... I believe it was dated 1918, 1919, something like that. It was one dollar, where the doctor had made a house call. It was one dollar. Otherwise, I don't know. We were young and not concerned with the price of it, but I don't know that they [doctors] weren't paid. I don't imagine it was an exorbitant rate. If it would have been, we couldn't have afforded them[66]

Martha Ferguson's oldest two children were born at home in 1937 and 1938. She recalled, "The doctor and the nurse came for $25 and they stayed the entire time. Jim — no, David — was born in the country [in 1944].... The doctor came at that time too, but

I'm not sure how much that cost. It was a lot more than $25."[67]

Few respondents remembered having medical insurance before the 1950s. Doctor's bills were paid out of pocket. When asked how people paid for their health care services when he was young, Richard Finfgeld responded:

> I suppose they sent you a bill. I don't know. My father's principal objective was to see that every bill was paid. So he would ask them what the bill was and pay it. When we came here to Henry, I went in to see Dr. Dicer down here when I had a cold or something. I asked him how much it was for the visit and he said, "A half a dollar." And I paid him. So maybe they paid that way.[68]

Only Martha Ferguson, who worked for General Electric in Morton for almost thirty years beginning in the 1950s, remembered group health insurance, saying, "You had to pay for the family card which didn't cost that much, and I did pay for it."[69]

Even after World War II, the cost of medical care was generally viewed as reasonable and affordable. Margaret Esposito's husband, a career military officer, suffered from lung cancer in the late 1950s. He became ill when the family was living in Arizona, and they returned to Bloomington where he was cared for in Margaret's family home:

> The doctor would come out to the house. And I must say he was good about that. And he was especially good since the military would not release any medical records.
> *Interviewer*: Did the military pay for your husband's medical treatment?
> *Respondent*: All the medical treatment that was done, and I could take him over to Chanute any time, and then they did put him in a couple of times down at Scott for x-ray therapy to relieve the pain. But as far as paying for, I don't think they, I could get the medications from them. But I don't think they paid the doctor bill. I think that was an insignificant amount.
> *Interviewer*: Was it?
> *Respondent*: And we just paid. . . . Yeah.
> *Interviewer*: Did you have health insurance aside from what you had through the military?
> *Respondent*: No.[70]

Several respondents commented on the increase in health care costs. One woman born in 1966 had her babies in 1989 and 1991. She remembered:

> Oh, the doctor for Daniel — it was $1200 for a vaginal delivery and $1400 for a c-section. For Molly, it was $1475 for a vaginal and $1600 for a c-section. So it increased some $200 within those two years. For the hospital — both times I was in the hospital in those two years — it was $250 a day per mother and per child. $1000 for two days in the hospital. For Daniel a lot of it was paid for. I really don't know what the costs were. We only had to pay $25 to the hospital, and then we had to pay some of the blood-work. . . . For Molly, I had a $250 deductible, so I paid for my bloodwork and my ultrasound. . . . But we got lucky, because St. Francis, since we were in a lower tax bracket, they picked up the tab. The Sisters of St. Francis had a fund for people with insurance but have a big amount left over to pay. We only paid $500 for Molly. We were lucky with both of them really. A lot of people have complications and stay in the hospital longer and have a bigger bill. Rhonda, she was in premature labor from the time she was three or four months pregnant with Shelby. So she had a home contraction monitor, which cost. She was in the hospital two weeks before she had her. She thought she was going to have her, and they wouldn't let her have her, and then they gave her a shot to develop her lungs, and then a week and a half later she finally went and did have her. So she had a hospital stay previous to when she had her. So her bills were easily $10,000 with insurance. They are still paying on that.[71]

These comments reveal more than a natural inflation in charges for medical services. They indicate that the services themselves have changed. Technologically-dependent health care delivered in institutional settings is expensive compared to advice and service given in patients' homes. In addition, modern expectations of health care demand miraculous interventions, which come with a hefty price tag.

Birth

The management of pregnancy and childbirth has changed

dramatically during the twentieth century. Before about 1920, pregnancy, although regarded as a special condition, was a private and personal matter, concealed if possible and certainly not considered a medical condition requiring a physician's supervision. Older oral history respondents did not remember their mothers receiving any prenatal care from medical practitioners. Indeed, Grace Allman said, "I don't think she [mother] ever saw a doctor until he came to deliver the baby."[72] Regular visits to the doctor during pregnancy became common at about the same time as hospital delivery — between about 1920 and 1940.

The environment and management of childbirth have also changed significantly. Home deliveries, usual before the 1930s, occurred in the familiar domestic setting, largely controlled by the mother and her family. Although professional experts, including physicians, midwives, and nurses, supervised the birth process, interventions such as the use of anesthetics, instruments and surgery were less common than they became when childbirth moved into hospitals.

This move was welcomed by both doctors and patients for a number of reasons. Physicians increasingly viewed childbirth as a pathological process, fraught with dangers to mother and infant. In an influential article published in 1920, Dr. Joseph DeLee of Chicago described the hazards of unaided birth:

> So frequent are these bad effects, that I have often wondered whether Nature did not deliberately intend women to be used up in the process of reproduction, in a manner analogous to that of the salmon, which dies after spawning.[73]

He advocated the use of forceps and episiotomy in normal birth to protect both mother and baby from injury. In hospitals, these routine interventions could be more conveniently administered. In addition, the hospital environment offered resources useful in the event of the complications which could arise even in apparently normal births. For example, as hospital utilization grew, the number of caesarean sections performed increased. Although increased levels of intervention did not, in the first half of the twentieth century, reduce maternal or infant mortality, both doctors and lay people became convinced that hospitals offered a kind of insurance against the hazards of childbirth.

Women were easily persuaded that hospital delivery was safer and more convenient than home birth. Hospitals were increasingly seen as germ-free compared to homes, thus providing a sanitary environment for both mothers and babies. In addition, hospitals were especially equipped to deal with the mess of birth, while homes were not. Hospitals were also more likely to offer an increasing range of anesthetics and pain-relieving drugs, which were welcomed by women as modern weapons against the discomfort of labor and delivery.[74]

With the move from home to hospital, childbirth was increasingly dealt with as a medical problem. Accomplished in an environment controlled by institutional regulations and procedures, birth was increasingly managed by medical personnel and separated from ordinary social and family life. In addition, general experience of labor and birth changed with routine use of a growing range of interventions. According to one authority:

> Medicine . . . continued to emphasize efficiency and speed in labor and delivery, objectives that many women shared. The obstetric comparison between the automobile assembly line and the mother was not without relevance. Nor was the comparison of the mother to a broken-down automobile and the hospital to an automobile maintenance and repair shop. During the 1940s, 1950s and 1960s, birth was the processing of a machine by machines and skilled technicians.[75]

The development of a range of new diagnostic and monitoring technologies in the second half of the twentieth century further increased mothers' dependence on professional medicine. Not until the 1970s did parents begin to seek a more active role in the birth process by embracing the use of 'natural childbirth' techniques such as Lamaze and demanding involvement in both decisions made about how deliveries were managed and environments in which they took place.

Oral history interviews illustrate changes in the management of childbearing which have occurred in living memory. They trace the transition from traditional home birth to hospital delivery. They also demonstrate changes in expectations and costs associated with childbearing.

In the past, the circumstances and management of birth were closely related to the parents' culture. Alice Swift, born in 1927, grew up in an Amish Mennonite community which adhered to traditional European ways of dealing with childbirth. Her mother remembered having worked before her own marriage by doing:

Housework as well as taking care of mothers with new babies in their homes.

Interviewer: Was this part of a church role that was customary?

Respondent: Yes. It was a customary pattern for single women to do this. Women in those days did not go to the hospital, in our particular group at least, so they always had their babies at home. . . .

Interviewer: Did she actually assist during the childbirth?

Respondent: Possibly, but not as a midwife particularly; just to be there to take care of the baby.[76]

Mrs. Rittenhouse, born into a Mennonite family in 1941, remembered rendering similar services to her mother's sisters when she was a teenager:

I know as a young child or as a young teenager — real young teenager, 12 or 13 — I would go to her [mother's] sisters and help after they had their children and stay for a week or two. And just help with the chores and stuff like that. . . . I helped with the dishes and scrubbed floors and that sort of thing. I didn't do too much with the baby. . . . I did that for my Aunt Darlene at least twice and my Aunt Florence once. And I would go and stay with them. One lived in Streator and the other lived in Champaign.[77]

It is likely that these traditional services served the dual functions of providing useful help to the newly delivered mother and educating young women about their future role.

Mrs. Rueger, a Mennonite born in 1913, said that, in addition to the local physician, her paternal aunt and a midwife, who was also a friend of the family, were present at her own birth:

Of course then you see, as you called the midwife, she stayed for ten days and she would do cooking and everything.

Interviewer: She would take care of the baby?

Respondent: Yes.[78]

This respondent was cared for by the same midwife when she gave birth to her second child in the 1930s. As had become common by this time, she went to her doctor for monthly check-ups during her pregnancy; then, when her labor began, she called the midwife:

I . . . had her spoken for to come when the baby came. That was the way we did it. She knew and would call the doctor and say, "Well, now, you better come pretty soon."
Interviewer: So the midwife notified the doctor then. Did you have a telephone at that time?
Respondent: Oh, yeah. . . . We were at Harold's parents that evening until about 10 o'clock, I guess, and came home, and I could not get comfortable. Pretty soon we thought that this was it. So we made the telephone call so my mom would bring out the midwife. And Bill was there at 8 o'clock. . . .
Interviewer: . . . During the actual labor or delivery part of it, did the doctor use any kind of instruments? Medicine?
Respondent: No. At one time he thought he might need to, so he told the midwife to put on water to boil. But we didn't need it. And I had no medication.
Interviewer: What would they have used the water for?
Respondent: Instruments — sterilize them.[79]

Before the 1930s, it was usual for members of all social groups, rural and urban, to give birth at home, and for female family members, friends or paid workers to be present to offer both moral support and help with household duties. Grace Allman, born in a rural community in 1896, said:

All five of my mother's children were born at home.
Interviewer: Do you know who delivered?
Respondent: Dr. Wright.
Interviewer: Was anyone else present at the birth?
Respondent: Yes. There was a woman who came and stayed with her, kept her in bed for ten days.
Interviewer: Do you know who that woman was?
Respondent: No, sir. We all had different women. I don't know the woman who was there when my brothers were born, but I know the one who was there when my sisters were born; her name was Mrs. Morris, Alice Morris. The last . . . [nurse] was Rachel Wright, and my sister was named for that nurse — Rachel.[80]

Ruth Carpenter, born on a farm in 1909, said of her own mother:

She had all of her babies at home. And we had a lady in the neighborhood that was what we'd call a midwife. Only she wasn't certified of course. But she did a lot of it and she never had any problems.[81]

Lucinda Brent Posey, born in Streator in 1914, remembered:

> Nothing [about sex and reproduction] was explained by my mother. However, she had a book hidden in her trunk that I read. My sister-in-law taught me the facts of life, about babies, etc. Aunt Lucy Dabney had nine children, all delivered at home. My mother would be called to come. I had to go with her, so I learned a lot from listening to conversations.[82]

Dorothy Jean Stewart, said of her own birth in Bloomington in 1933:

> I was born at home in the dining room. Dr. Brown delivered me, and I understand that Elizabeth Johnson, a native of Bloomington, also assisted in the birth. I suppose they were so busy watching the second coming of me that they almost put the ether in my mother's eyes instead of to her nose.[83]

This account is interesting because anesthetic was used for this home delivery.

While birth was regarded as the natural and expected role of women, it was also considered dangerous. Ruth Carpenter remembered that when she was young, "Mother mortality was terrific."[84] Thus, birth was not an experience all women wanted. Marie Bostic, born in 1897, said about childbearing, "That's one thing I never wanted. . . . I saw a couple of them, but I said I hope that never happens to me. He [husband] said, "We'll do what we can to keep you from it."[85] The Bostics remained childless.

Because childbirth was regarded as a life threatening experience, in the early years of the twentieth century new mothers stayed in bed for a long time; oral history respondents recalled the standard period of convalescence being between ten days and two weeks. Getting up too soon after delivery was believed to be dangerous. Ruth Carpenter remembered, "And I knew a lady . . . well, it'd be my cousin's wife, and she died from a hemorrhage from getting up postpartum."[86] Thus, it was usual for either female family members or paid nurses to stay in the household to do housework and look after younger children. Sometimes, alternatively, children were sent to stay with relatives during their mother's confinement. Grace Allman recalled:

I have a scar on my hand here that doesn't show too much any more, but it used to stand up permanently because when my first brother was born, I was a year and a half old so they took me out in the country to live with my aunt until Mother was up and around again. As my father was bringing me home in the buggy, I began to cry. He didn't know what was the matter with me because I had been good all the way home, but I cried. When they got me inside and began to unwrap me, there was a blister. He had been smoking a cigar and some of the ashes fell on my hand and made a blister there. It made a scar....

Interviewer: After your mother had a baby, do you know if any relatives stayed around to help her?

Respondent: No, but they had a hired girl that came and helped her. It was a woman who lived next door to us who came and worked there. She got $3 a week.[87]

In the 1930s, pregnancy and birth were becoming increasingly "medicalized." Oral history respondents who gave birth during or after that decade remembered receiving regular medical care during their pregnancies.[88] However, before the 1960s most consulted general practitioners, rather than obstetricians. Mrs. Rittenhouse remembered:

Well, at that time people went to their family doctors, whether they were having children, stomachache or headache or whatever. The family doctor took care of it, so I suppose some people at that time may have gone to an obstetrician, but I didn't and didn't even think about it at the time.[89]

Hospital delivery was increasingly seen as an alternative to home birth by both urban and rural women, although many customs surrounding confinement, including long periods in bed, remained. According to Caribel Washington, whose son was born in 1935:

I went dancing two weeks before he was [supposed to be] born. He wasn't supposed to be born in January, he was supposed to be born in February. So they had a big dance. This used to be a nice dance time and I loved to dance. So we went dancing and my doctor was there and he said, "Will you go and sit down in a chair, please, until they play their final song?" I said, "Why? I feel fine!" ... Then when

I got home that night I began to have a bit of a stom-achache and I though, "Oh, I shouldn't have ate some raw oysters over there, that's what's making me sick!" Eleven o'clock the next morning, there was a baby! . . . I hardly got to the hospital. I never even got to the delivery room. I can't even tell you where the delivery room is. He just came. That was it!

Interviewer: . . . You did go to the hospital though?

Respondent: The doctor was in the cab with me. That's why he was there. . . . He [husband] just walked over and told the doctor I was sick and the doctor came over. He told my husband, "Well, you better get a cab." He and I went to the hospital and that's how he helped me deliver!

Interviewer: Okay. Do you remember how long you had to stay?

Respondent: Yes! I had to stay 13 days, which I felt was ridiculous! Absolutely ridiculous! But that's when they believed women ought to stay in the hospital for two weeks.[90]

Margaret Esposito's daughter was born in 1947. Esposito was attended by an obstetrician, Dr. O.H. Ball, and her delivery was more managed than was typical of older respondents:

I had a breech presentation with my daughter. A very diffi-cult time. . . .

Interviewer: Did you have any anesthetic when you had your daughter?

Respondent: Only for the last little bit . . . to kind of give me some pain relief. And I had an extensive episiotomy. Because she also had the cord around the neck. And so I know I wasn't any cooperation to him [doctor]. He had to do it . . . . I was something. I'm sure he was pretty upset with me. Because I would not have a spinal.[91]

Birth in the hospital environment was different in many ways from home births. At home, although the doctor was respon-sible for technical matters, the environment was controlled by the mother. By and large, she decided who was present at the birth and who could see and handle the newborn. Increasingly strict hospital regulations and procedures altered both the physical and the social environment of childbirth. Ruth Carpenter, who began nursing in the 1930s, said that at the beginning of her career, newborns were not isolated in nurseries:

> In those days, we had a cart, and they had a pan around
> the cart about that high and you could lay babies crosswise,
> and that cart would hold eight babies. Yeah. And we'd
> take 'em over in the middle building [at Brokaw]. And I
> know. . . . Especially on Saturday and Sunday, when people
> would flock in like bees on honey, and . . . I bet there wasn't
> a baby on them carts that didn't get kissed.
> *Interviewer*: So you weren't as worried about the germs
> then.
> *Respondent*: No. We didn't worry about it.
> *Interviewer*: Well, did you let the other family members
> come in. You know, dads and grandparents and other chil-
> dren in the family?
> *Respondent*: Yeah. Everybody could. Yeah. They could
> come in. . . and see 'em.
> *Interviewer*: So when did they change that rule, then. . . ?
> *Respondent*: It got pretty strict. . . . In 1940 I had an OB
> case that had a C-section, and they became part of my fam-
> ily sort of. And I brought the baby down from surgery and
> the father was waiting at the elevator for him and I let him
> look at that baby and the supervisor like to had a fit.
> *Interviewer*: Really?
> *Respondent*: I said, "Well, it's his baby. If he can't look at
> it, I don't know why."[92]

Hospitals also made rules about who could be present in
the delivery room, often banning all family members. Ralph
Spencer's daughter was born at Mennonite Hospital in 1936. He
remembered:

> Well, my wife's mother was with me. We were there, but
> we weren't. . . my wife's mother was not in the delivery
> room. I was.
> *Interviewer*: Oh you were? That was unusual for that
> time.
> *Respondent*: Well, I'll tell ya, I and the head nurse there at
> Mennonite, you wouldn't know who she was, her name was
> Maxwell. She was the head of that thing. . . . When my
> wife went in for delivery, she said, "I want my husband
> with me." The nurse said, "Yeah, sure, sure, sure." I stood
> out in the hallway and waited, and when nobody showed

up, I just opened the door and went in. Maxwell was there and she said, "You can't come in here!" I said, "Well, I'm in here." "You can't come in here without a cap and gown on!" I told her she better get one because I wasn't going anywhere. And I did. I stayed right there when the baby was born.[93]

Margaret Esposito's husband was also present for the births of their children in the late 1940s at the recommendation of Dr. Ball, who wanted fathers in the delivery room despite what he perceived to be the nurses' objections.[94]

By the 1960s, hospital management of birth became as regulated as it would ever be. When Mrs. Rittenhouse's first child was born in 1961, she called her parents to tell them she and her husband were going to the hospital. Her parents stayed at home because, "They couldn't come in anyway, so nobody came over. Bill [husband] was there, and that was it." She went on to say:

Nobody else was allowed on the delivery floor. Nobody was allowed in the delivery room. Even Bill wasn't allowed in the delivery room. He was just allowed in the labor room, and the parents weren't allowed to come in anyway.[95]

In the 1970s, things began to change in response to women's interest in taking a more active role in the birth process. Sally Wagner, an obstetrical nurse, began to teach Lamaze classes in Bloomington in 1972. She said:

At first, . . . the doctors were real skeptical about Lamaze. They were used to heavily sedating patients and the patients were not active in their labor process. They were very passive because they were sedated heavily. The doctors were really negative — how could this possibly work? They definitely did not feel like the fathers belonged in the delivery room, and so that was a big battle. . . . They thought that they would get sick, faint, or sue the doctor. . . . It took awhile to get them convinced and now they do let them go in for c-sections and so forth and it took a few years to convince them that it was okay to let them in for an operation. We've come a long ways and the doctors are very positive.[96]

Mrs. Rohm's two children were born in 1989 and 1991.

While her pregnancies and deliveries were medically monitored to a much greater degree than those of older respondents, she was much more actively involved in the process than they had been. She and her husband used Lamaze techniques, enhanced by pain relieving drugs, during her deliveries. She also asked her doctor for information about management of her care:

> What did I ask him? Oh, there was a little mixup as to when my due date was. And I had a lot of blood work done, and I would ask them why I had to do that. And what their procedures — how they handle things in the hospital, when to call . . . them, how far apart your contractions need to be before you get ahold of the doctor, and how you go about these things. . . . I thought I had gall stones with Daniel, and I asked him about that and had an ultrasound for that. But I knew most other things. I would ask Wendy [sister] first, before I asked the doctor.[97]

This example illustrates women's enduring reliance on adult female family members, which transcends the medicalization of reproduction. It also illustrates the late twentieth-century trend for women to learn as much as possible about pregnancy, delivery, and medical management of these processes in order to make intelligent decisions regarding their own treatment and get the childbirth experiences they desire.

Health Care and Race

There have been African American residents in McLean County since its establishment. In 1900, this group comprised approximately two percent of the County's population. Although not subjected to the legally sanctioned segregation usual in the American South of the early twentieth century, McLean County's African Americans suffered from discrimination affecting the opportunities and quality of life available to them. For example, Reginald Whitaker's father had received a college degree in business as a young man. However, he was never employed at the professional level for which he was qualified. "There was nothing for an Afro-American in Business Administration." Thus, his father worked at a laundry for over twenty years and finished his working life as a janitor in the Livingston Building in downtown Bloomington. When asked if his father felt frustrated by his limited career opportunities, Mr. Whitaker said, "No. He understood the period of the time and I guess there was no point in being frustrated. Things were like they were then."[98]

Things were also "like they were then" in areas other than employment. Although African Americans were able to attend Illinois State Normal University in the mid-twentieth century, they did so under conditions different from those of their white colleagues. According to Beulah Kennedy, born in the 1920s, "When I was coming up and going to school at ISNU, it was very discriminatory. You couldn't live on campus. You had to live in somebody's private home. Of course, I didn't have that problem because I was at home."[99] While African Americans began to be admitted to local nursing schools in the 1950s, they also had to find accommodation outside of the residence halls.[100]

African Americans were able to obtain professional medical care in McLean County, both from white physicians and from the few black doctors who settled in Bloomington. Caribel Washington, born in 1914, remembered:

> Oh, yes. We had doctors all the time. We had Dr. Covington who was an African-American doctor. A very good doctor. I can recall my mother's doctor was Dr. Greenleaf. . . . Then there was always Dr. Brown and Dr. McNutt. Those were the two doctors for the most part who doctored the African-American people. There might have been others. . . . I don't say there weren't others, but I do know that those two seemed to be the main doctors back in the '20s and maybe the early '30s. Of course, with the Depression, we had another [black] doctor, but he had no business during the Depression because we had no money. But there were always doctors for the people.[101]

Oscar Waddell, born in 1917, remembered his family's relationship with their physician:

> And back in those days, we had a Negro doctor here.
> *Interviewer*: Was that Dr. Covington?
> *Respondent*: Yes, that was Dr. Covington. But Dr. Fenelon took care of us boys. Dr. Fenelon would always call and want us to come up and get a shot. He was on the sixth floor of the Greisham Building. The building that burned. We would go up there; here were two little black boys come in there. And the nurse would say, "Yes, Mrs. Waddell, the doctor has been expecting you." The doctor would come

out, "Oh, what do we have here? Come on in! Bring my boys on in here!" I would ask, "What are you going to do, Doc?" He would say, "Come on in here, I got some candy for you." You would hear them [other patients] say, "How come they get in ahead of us?" The doctor would give us a shot and tell our mother. . . , "They are getting this for diphtheria." And everything that came up, we would get a shot. He would tell her what to do. Back in those days, Dad never bought us any Easter, Fourth of July or anything. The Doc would always get that.[102]

While white physicians apparently did not discriminate against African-American patients, they were less tolerant of black doctors. Dr. Eugene Covington was apparently the only African American physician to have received full privileges in local hospitals before World War II. According to Lucinda Brent Posey, Dr. W.B. Hatcher, who graduated from Meharry Medical College, a traditionally black medical school, in 1923, "Practiced at hospitals, but without full privileges, meaning that a full privilege physician had to okay his orders."[103]

Like other African-American respondents, Reginald Whitaker recalled that his family had ready access to care from physicians, both general practitioners and specialists. However, obtaining dental care was more problematical:

Interviewer: Did you go to the dentist?
Respondent: That was a problem. No. Not until recent years. They wouldn't accept you. They had one black dentist here years ago, his name was Thompson, I think. I don't know how long he stayed here. He had an office uptown somewhere, downtown Bloomington, I should say. We just didn't go to the dentist. . . .
Interviewer: Now, why do you suppose there was such a difference between doctors and dentists? You said the doctors didn't make any difference.
Respondent: Well, I don't know. . . . It's hard to explain prejudice. . . . Maybe a doctor is examining, putting that stethoscope on you and listening to your heart and lungs, diagnosing your problem. A dentist has got to go into your mouth with his instruments and what-have-you. I guess a black person's mouth was contaminated to them or something. I don't know.[104]

African Americans also encountered discrimination in medical institutions. For example, Fairview Sanitarium did not house black patients in the main building during the years before World War II; rather, they had separate accommodation. According to Caribel Washington:

> Well, of course we were always afraid of tuberculosis. And I think probably after the Sanitarium came on, people had such an abhorrence to it because the African Americans couldn't stay in the Sanitarium. They had a little place outside where they stayed.[105]

Some local hospitals also discriminated against African Americans. According to Lucinda Brent Posey:

> At Brokaw, a black patient was put in a room wherever there was an empty bed, regardless of color. This was in the early 1940s I know about. At St. Joseph's Hospital, two blacks were always put into the same room or a room by yourself. If they couldn't do this, the response was "no beds". Regardless of how much moving around was necessary, one never was in a room with a white person — until integration.

Mrs. Posey herself became Brokaw hospital's second black employee in 1943 when she was hired as Medical Record Administrator. The first was Elizabeth Brent Keyes who went to work in the laundry in 1915.[106]

Since the 1960s, discrimination in health care provision on the basis of race has declined. Non-white residents of McLean County have, at least theoretically, the same ability to obtain medical, dental and hospital treatment as their white neighbors. However, since disproportionate numbers of African Americans live in poverty, economic barriers, particularly among the working poor, have replaced racial discrimination in inhibiting access to a full range of high quality health care services for many blacks.

Death

During the twentieth century, management of death, like illness and childbearing, was increasingly professionalized and institutionalized. Early in the century, traditional ways of dealing with the end of life survived. The dying were cared for at home by relatives and neighbors. Bodies were prepared for burial by lay-people who exercised skills learned by attendance at many death-beds as a voluntary community service for which they did not expect to be paid. Relatives, friends, and neighbors sat up all night with the recently deceased in wakes rendering respect to the bereaved family and offering an informal opportunity for collective grief. Organizing funerals was the responsibility of family and church members.[107]

By 1900, however, things had already begun to change. It had become usual, particularly in larger towns, for trained under-takers to deal with the mechanical aspects of death. They pre-pared bodies for burial, first in private homes, later in specially equipped funeral homes or parlors. They began to offer embalm-ing — a procedure which could only be performed by experts. They supplied coffins and organized funerals. While providing a wel-come service, increasingly professional undertakers, now also referred to as morticians and funeral directors, also developed a business opportunity for which there was a steady market. The oral history interviews conducted for this project illustrate nation-al trends in the management of dying and death.

Older respondents recalled that death almost always occurred at home. It was usual for the terminally ill to be cared for by relatives. Martha Ferguson's grandmother died during the 1930s. She commented, "It was common to take care of a dying person in the home. My mother took care of my grandmother; it was just common." This is not to say that performing this service was easy. Mrs. Ferguson said, "I do know that she had breast can-cer. In those days they didn't know much about cancer. She thought she got it from falling downstairs and injuring herself. My mother had a lingering hard time with my grandmother going."[108]

It remained usual for sufferers from chronic degenerative diseases to be cared for at home in the second half of the twentieth century, even after other serious health problems had moved into the hospital. Several respondents described caring for relatives suffering from Alzheimer's Disease and cancer in the years between 1950 and 1980, receiving increasing support from health care providers and other service agencies.[109] However, even the acutely ill and seriously injured were nursed at home in the days before speedy ambulance service and easily accessible hospital emergency rooms. Marie Bostic, born in 1897, remembered her great grandmother's death in about 1908:

My great grandmother who lived in town here, she was the greatest thing. I can remember her just like it was yesterday. They had one of these round stoves, you know. . . of course, you'd never see her legs because they had long dresses. She used goose grease and kerosene, and she got her clothes saturated with that, you know, and was burned. . . . She lived alone. She got up and somewhere or other she turned around, and her dress tail got in that fire. It went up her back, and I guess she was really something else.

Interviewer: That's terrible!

Respondent: Yes it was. She screamed and the boys from the restaurant heard her. . . and they got burned. . . . Threw her on the ground, wrapped her up, and got her to the doctor. She burned on Tuesday. She died on Friday. She was buried on Sunday. Easter Sunday. She always went to church on Easter. She went to church, but she went in a coffin. . . .

Interviewer: Was she taken to a funeral home?

Respondent: No. . . . It was all done at home.[110]

As this interview indicates, in the early twentieth century it was also usual for bodies to be prepared for burial at home, and kept at home until the funeral. Older respondents — particularly those from rural communities — remembered "laying out" being a voluntary service rather than a profession or business operation. Grace Allman's grandfather died in about 1914. She said that "They didn't have funeral homes in those days", so the body was prepared for burial by Mr. F.L. Garst. When asked whether Mr. Garst performed this service for other people in the community, Mrs. Allman said, "I don't know. He really was a banker. That was sort of a side issue." As far as she knew, Mr. Garst was not paid for his help.[111] Grace Allman also remembered members of the community sitting up with the recently deceased during the nights before the funeral:

Interviewer: What was the reasoning for staying up with a dead person?

Respondent: Well, I'll tell ya. Before they embalmed bodies they had to keep it as cool as they could and they did it with cool cloths and things of that kind that they would put over their faces, you know. It was sort of necessary then, but it became unnecessary, of course.[112]

Ralph Spencer also participated in wakes, which he defined as follows: "A wake is where a person is dead and two or three people sit up all night during the night. I have done that."[113]

By this time, voluntary private management of death was increasingly old-fashioned even in rural communities. More common was the paid undertaker who visited the homes of the recently deceased to prepare bodies for burial. Ralph Spencer's grandparents died at home within two months of each other in about 1920. He said:

> I don't know if there was a funeral home in existence at that time or not.
> *Interviewer*: Then the bodies were probably cared for at home then?
> *Respondent*: They were cared for at home, right. . . . A reason why I know who the funeral personnel was was the fact that at that time it was in the spring of the year and the roads had thawed out and they had to use a horse hearse. That was the only horse hearse that was around. Mr. Otto had a horse hearse. He had a farmer out here with a big team of horses to pull that hearse. That's how I knew. Of course, knowing Otto from the time I was a little kid on, I knew he took care of my grandparents and then I knew him from then on till the time he died. You just don't forget those things either, see.
> *Interviewer*: So this same person performed this type of service for other people in the community?
> *Respondent*: Yes. He was the only mortician there was around locally. They had them in Bloomington — Becks, but I think Becks was the only one at that time.
> *Interviewer*: Do you know if Otto was compensated in any way for performing this service?
> *Respondent*: Oh sure. . . . I know he was compensated monetarily, yes.[114]

Marie Bostic remembered a series of undertakers serving the population of Danvers, beginning with a Mr. Lowe who looked after her grandmother.[115]

By the mid-twentieth century, death was managed by professionals. People more frequently died in hospitals or nursing homes. Preparation of the body and funeral arrangements were performed by trained and licensed experts. When asked about changes in death and dying since her youth, Martha Ferguson said, "I think it is nice that the body goes to the funeral home instead of the home now. It's just easier for the family to go through it that way." This change came with a price tag. All aspects of the process became more costly[116] In addition, death, like birth and illness, became increasingly remote from ordinary experience. Recognition and expression of grief was no longer expected, or even considered to be good manners. Mrs. Ferguson commented, "Nobody wears mourning. Then [in the past] they would go in black and wear it for a year or whatever. Nobody does that." [117] Grace Allman remembered a much more emotional response to death in the past:

> My folks used to live across from the Presbyterian Church over there and we've had people come out of that church and just cry until you could hear them yell clear across the street, the way that they were crying and going on. Nobody does that anymore. . . . I think people have more control over their emotions than they used to. I think they shed lots of tears at home, but they try to hold up in public.[118]

Perhaps in an age when ordinary people are not expected to do anything about dying and death, they have become less able to view these experiences as the inevitable consequence of life — as universal as birth.

Conclusions

This chapter uses oral history evidence to illustrate changes in the ways McLean County residents have experienced illness, medical care, birth, and death during the twentieth century. This evidence indicates that local experience reflects national trends. Popularization of the germ theory and development of drugs effective in preventing and curing infectious diseases transformed both the range of ailments threatening people and the treatment of these ailments. Infant and child mortality declined; expectations regarding the duration and quality of life increased. Disease and death were increasingly associated with old age. The triumphs of medical science and public health which underlay these developments also supported significant changes in the management of birth, illness and death.

The twentieth century is the age of the expert. Amateur management of birth, illness, and death is considered, at best, uninformed; at worst, illegal. In living memory, all of these processes have moved out of private homes into institutions. Lay people gratefully relinquish responsibility for them to professionals. Because of expanding market demand, institutionally-based professional health care and funeral services have become lucrative businesses, generating still more business activity in the form of a range of financial and support services. As business transactions, they stray from the traditional context for personal care. The challenge for the next century will be to rationalize the expectations, services and costs of health care without sacrificing the personal relationships which are so important in meeting the real needs of sufferers and healers. Perhaps community health care planning can benefit from an understanding of historical experience.

Conclusion: The Face in the Mirror

The history of health, illness and medicine is about all of us. It is about the anticipation of birth; the worry over the sick-bed of a beloved child; the impotence attending the decline of an elderly parent; the fear of dying; the finality of death. It is about how we feel and what we do. It is about where and when we live. It is about our mortality and our ingenuity — those elements which define our humanity.

This book has argued that the experience of McLean County residents during the past 160 years has illustrated national trends. The communities, neighborhoods, health care providers and individuals of this midwestern American county reflect the sweeping changes in health, illness and medical care which have occurred elsewhere in the United States and, indeed, the developed world. The most significant of these changes concern developments in public health and sanitation; the institutionalization of health care; professionalization and specialization among health care providers; and, finally, the rising expectations and costs of medical treatment which, in the last quarter of the twentieth century, have generated what many view to be a crisis in health care delivery.

Public Health and Sanitation

Perhaps the least dramatic, but most significant, changes during the period covered by this study have been the gradual improvements in general living standards and expectations regarding the quality and length of life which are reflected in both the environment and the individuals who occupy it. These improvements depend upon developments which are so generally taken for granted that they have attained almost the status of natural phenomena — drained agricultural fields, indoor plumbing, drinkable tap water, pasteurized milk, inspected meat, garbage collection. In McLean County, as elsewhere, these developments evolved for a variety of reasons which were not necessarily related to modern understanding of disease causation. For example, fields were drained, not for health but for logistical and economic reasons; soggy fields were harder to plow and less productive than dry ones. Nonetheless, the coincidental eradication of malaria-

235

bearing mosquitoes improved the health of County residents and made the area more attractive to new migrants in the second half of the nineteenth century.

Developments in sanitation depended upon changing theories about the causes of diseases. Early street paving schemes, sewerage systems, and garbage collection services were predicated on an assumed cause-effect relationship between dirt and illness. Nineteenth-century urban reformers and sanitarians believed that accumulated filth produced the *miasma*, or polluted atmosphere, which generated a host of ailments ranging from malaria to cholera. Thus, towns began clean-up campaigns which improved the health of their citizens long before general acceptance of the germ theory. The earliest urban center of McLean County, Bloomington, began health-related civic improvements in the 1870s which would be mirrored in other settlements as they grew.

Prevention campaigns became more precise and effective after the popularization of the germ theory around the turn of the twentieth century. Sources of contagion could be clearly identified; procedures preventing infection could be specified and followed. McLean County residents became accustomed to legal regulation of their behavior for the purpose of curbing the spread of certain diseases. Quarantine signs protected the healthy from the ailing; by the mid-twentieth century, proof of immunization was required for school attendance. Beginning in the early 1900s, milk and meat could be laboratory tested for disease-producing organisms; with the establishment of the County Health Department in 1945, inspection and testing were routinely done.

In addition to its impact on civic life, the popularization of the germ theory transformed individuals' relationships with the environment. Early twentieth-century housewives scoured their homes, not merely for aesthetic or status reasons, but to hold at bay the invisible army of microbes threatening their families. Mothers learned that boiling baby bottles reduced the danger of the diarrheas which had killed so many infants in the past. Children were taught to cover their mouths when they coughed or sneezed; to wash their hands after going to the toilet; and to take frequent baths as a way of protecting both themselves and others from disease-bearing germs. Once its connection to tuberculosis was established, public spitting became illegal in many communities. Thus, in the twentieth century personal hygiene gained both a scientific rationale and an increased status which projected it beyond good manners and personal fastidiousness into moral imperative and social responsibility.

236

These private and collective measures taken to prevent illness have had a tremendous impact on the duration and quality of life. More than medical therapies, they have altered the range of diseases people most fear, and those they are most likely to die of. In the nineteenth century, McLean County residents succumbed to infectious illnesses long before they were old enough to develop the cardiovascular diseases and cancers which most frequently kill their twentieth-century descendants. A century ago, it was considered normal, though sad, for an infant or child to die; in the late twentieth century, such an event is as rare as it is tragic. Most communicable diseases can be either prevented by immunization or cured with antibiotics. Now McLean County residents, like other Americans, are increasingly faced with the challenges produced by success; they must find ways of preventing chronic ailments and caring for the growing numbers of frail elderly in their communities.

Institutionalization of Care

Before about 1920, most Americans were born, suffered illnesses, and died in their own homes. Physicians and nurses visited the ailing and applied treatments within domestic environments governed by householders. Doctor-patient relationships were analogous to those established between craftsmen and their clients; physicians were hired for their presumed expertise, but the ultimate responsibility for treatment decisions and day-to-day management remained with the adult relatives of sufferers. While doctors usually had offices, where they saw patients and dispensed medications, they spent most of their time making house calls.

Before the twentieth century, hospitals were relatively unimportant to most physicians' professional lives and figured not at all in most people's personal experience. McLean County's first charitable hospitals, St. Joseph's (established in 1880) and Deaconess/Brokaw (established in 1896), catered in early years to the poor and people without the appropriate resources for home care. While private sanitariums, such as Kelso's (built in 1894) offered comfortable facilities for rest and care to the prosperous, most of the well-heeled stayed home when they were ill, enjoying the personal attentions of physicians and private duty nurses.

The first half of the twentieth century witnessed dramatic changes in the environment of care. While continuing to make house calls, physicians began to encourage patients to visit their offices. With increasing urbanization, development of public transportation systems, and introduction of the automobile, it became less difficult for town-dwellers in particular to "go to the doctor's." With the introduction of new medical technology, such as x-ray machines and laboratory equipment used for diagnostic tests, physicians could offer a wider range of services in their offices. Furthermore, office care was more efficient and less stressful for the doctor, who could see more patients in less time and earn more money than was possible when delivering care to sufferers' homes. By the mid-twentieth century, it had become customary for town-dwellers to visit their doctors' offices under all but the most unusual circumstances. In the 1950s and '60s, rural residents joined this trend. By the last quarter of the century, house calls had virtually disappeared.

After 1900, in addition to office-based practice, hospital utilization also increased. The earliest type of medical treatment to be routinely institutionalized was surgery. With the development of first antiseptic, then aseptic surgical techniques, operations became safer and were performed more frequently. Hospital operating rooms were specially designed for surgical procedures; hospital environments were easier for medical personnel to control than patients' homes. Surgeons, who dominated hospital staffs and increasingly viewed hospitals as their professional homes, began to require their patients to be hospitalized as a matter of course. As certain kinds of minor surgery, including tonsillectomy and appendectomy, became routine, a growing number of people expected to be hospitalized at some point in their lives.

This number expanded as childbirth moved into hospitals after about 1920, when both physicians and patients began to regard the option of hospital delivery as a kind of insurance measure against complications which might occur during the birth process. Equipped with a range of technical and human resources not available in patients' homes, specialized hospital obstetrical facilities were marketed as safer, more convenient, and more comfortable than private homes. By 1940, virtually all babies born in McLean County were delivered in hospitals.

The range of conditions and numbers of patients treated in hospitals mushroomed with the introduction of antibiotics and an ever-expanding range of medical technologies after World War II. In the first half of the twentieth century, hospitals chiefly took pride in the provision of skilled nursing care. Patients rested, often for long periods of time, within the starched white environments which symbolized good hospital management. In the second half of the century, hospitals became veritable factories for the production of health. The duration of patient stays declined; the number of patients treated increased. Specialized types of equipment, found nowhere but hospitals, were applied to specific kinds of physical malfunctions; specialized technicians were trained to perform specific diagnostic and therapeutic procedures associated with increasingly standardized treatment programs.

Stimulated by government funding programs and popular demand, hospitals grew enormously in size and number. As they competed to attract patients, hospital environments became more luxurious and hospital care became more expensive. At the same time, hospital care was increasingly viewed as a necessity which must be afforded regardless of the expense. By the late twentieth century, virtually all births, serious illnesses and injuries were dealt with in hospitals.

The institutionalization of health care represents a dramatic break with the past. As ill-health moved out of private homes, people became increasingly helpless when confronted by it and increasingly dependent upon medical professionals. Witnesses of the impressive technology and miraculous achievements of modern medicine, they assumed that any health problem could be solved. At the same time, medical treatment became less personal than it had been in the days of home care. By the 1970s, popular resentment of professional institutional medicine became increasingly vocal.

Professionalization and Specialization

The nineteenth-century frontier doctor, who obtained most of his knowledge from the trial-and-error practice of medicine and carried all of his weapons against disease and injury in a small leather bag, is only a distant ancestor of his late twentieth-century descendants. In McLean County, as elsewhere, occupational medicine professionalized and specialized during the 160 years covered by this book.

Early members of the McLean County Medical Society worked in a diverse unregulated medical marketplace. A large variety of healers — trained and untrained; honest and fraudulent — competed for patients' loyalty and dollars. The main reasons for the establishment and operation of the Society were to impose order on and raise the standards of medical practice in the County. In addition, the organization protected the rights of its members and generated an *esprit de corps* which survived the changes of the twentieth century.

In 1900, virtually all physicians were general practitioners. The only specialization was informal and self-proclaimed. For example, some doctors deliberately developed surgical skills and did more surgery than their professional colleagues; however, formal board certification was still a generation away. Rapid developments in medical science, coupled with the establishment and growth of hospitals, however, fueled a trend in favor of specialization. Standardization of medical education, which by mid-century routinely included internships and residencies, created a formal structure for specialty training which was further supported by proliferation of examining boards.[1]

Specialists dominated the medical staffs of mid-twentieth-century hospitals. They dealt with serious health problems and performed dramatic interventions. As they became more effective in the struggle against disease and death, they demanded higher payment for their services. After World War II, in McLean County as elsewhere, specialists formed a growing elite among medical practitioners.

The trend toward specialization affected nursing as well. Nurses trained in the first half of the twentieth century developed general skills. Whether they worked as staff nurses in hospitals or did private duty nursing, they were expected to be able to provide basic care regardless of the kind of case assigned to them. Their training was largely based on observation and practice; there was little technology or theory for them to master.

Like medicine, nursing professionalized in the twentieth century. Under pressure from nursing organizations and demand for greater levels of skill from hospitals and physicians, nursing education became increasingly academic. Two- and three-year diploma programs, common in the early years of the century, gave way to degree programs after World War II. At the same time, hospitals began to employ graduate nurses who had developed the skills associated with new medical technology and new administrative paperwork. Nurses gained better working conditions, better wages and higher social and occupational status.

Following professional medicine, nursing also became increasingly specialized. Hospitals designated wards for specific categories of patients. Medical specialists demanded specialist skills from the nurses who assisted them. Nurses began to identify themselves, for example, as pediatric, obstetrical or surgical nurses.

Specialization among health care professionals developed in partnership with the institutionalization of care, raising similar concerns. Health care became more mechanized and less personal. While the patient gained access to a variety of experts, each extremely knowledgeable about a particular set of organs, disorders and therapies, s/he lost an environment of care which recognized the totality of the emotional, social and physical individual who suffers ill-health.

Rising Expectations and Costs

Memories of the days before miracle medicine are fading fast. Few now living can remember a time when the young routinely died of infections; when heart attacks were almost always fatal; when doctors were frequently helpless when faced with disease. Baby boomers cannot remember being without antibiotics; their children were born after the introduction of ultrasound examinations, CAT scans, and laser surgery.

Popular expectations of professional medicine have risen even more dramatically than its power against disease. Few illnesses are now assumed to be invariably fatal; the concept of natural death has almost disappeared. Lay-people believe that physicians can cure almost any disease — that if they find the right doctor who can apply the right treatment, health will be snatched from the jaws of death.

Along with rising expectations — indeed, because of them — the cost of medical care has skyrocketed. How much is a human life worth? How much is too much to pay for health? The terrified wife, the desperate father, the desolate child, responds that there is no price too high if one particularly precious life can be saved. While people deplore the growing bills for hospitalization, pharmaceutical drugs and doctors' care, they are also worried about the possibility of being deprived of these wonderful weapons against sickness and death. The development and widespread utilization of employer-based insurance plans after World War II blunted the impact of rising costs and ensured that growing numbers of people had access to medical care.

The profits associated with the provision of health care have turned hospitals, medical practices and health insurance companies into booming businesses. Bloomington-Normal, the urban medical center of McLean County, employs thousands of people in its health care organizations. Physicians flock to the area because of the local demand for their services; the institutional and technological resources available to them; and the comfortable lifestyle offered. Because the quality of care is high, both medical professionals and members of the wider community take pride in the County's health care delivery system.

However, in McLean County as elsewhere, the picture is not entirely rosy. The cost of health care, as a proportion of individual and national earnings, has risen to crisis proportions and is projected to rise still further. During the past quarter century, consumer advocates, politicians, and health care providers have posed the question of how our society can continue to pay for health care at current and projected rates. Various plans and policies have been proposed to address this issue. However, few have confronted the more significant and dangerous questions regarding what is being paid for; whether the prices charged are necessary or equitable; and whether all of the goods and services included in the cost of care are necessary to the treatment process.

The high price of health care has done more than lighten consumers' wallets. It has contributed to the trend favoring malpractice litigation. Because people expect to get what they pay for, they are disappointed and angry when medical care does not produce the desired result. Believing that physicians can perform miracles, patients feel cheated when their doctors make human mistakes. Beginning in the 1960s, County residents became increasingly willing to sue for malpractice. In response, health care providers began to insure themselves heavily and to practice increasingly defensive medicine. These developments further fueled the rise of health care costs. They also contributed to an erosion of the physician-patient relationship.

In addition, the rising expense of health care has limited access to it. While the Medicare and Medicaid legislation of the 1960s entitled many of McLean County's elderly and poor residents to certain kinds of care, other medical goods and services have remained prohibitively expensive. For example, senior citizens on fixed incomes must sometimes face the decision of whether to pay for food or prescription medicine, the cost of which is not covered by Medicare. Furthermore, increasing numbers of the working poor and self employed are without health insurance because it is so costly. Indeed, despite the national consensus that the number of people receiving public aid should be drastically reduced, loss of medical coverage associated with low-wage employment serves as a disincentive to work.

Into the Future

With other Americans, McLean County residents face inevitable changes in the way they obtain medical care. Managed

242

care has already arrived, and will almost certainly absorb most local health care providers and citizens because of its power to control costs and guarantee delivery of basic services. Because of its emphasis on the gatekeeping function of the primary care providers, there may be a trend away from proliferation of medical specialists and in favor of greater numbers of family doctors, physician assistants and nurse practitioners. Because of the high cost of hospitalization, in-patient care will probably continue to decline, while hospitals will provide an increasing range of out-patient, mobile and home-delivered services. Because of the expense of medical care in general, there will be a growing emphasis on health maintenance and disease prevention.

Superficially, these changes sound like a return to the good old days of general practitioners, house calls and hardy self reliance. However, there are significant differences between the remembered past and the health care of the future. Return to the days when access to professional medicine was regarded as a largely unnecessary luxury is impossible. Health care has become as necessary as secondary education and electricity. Thus, Americans must resolve the ongoing conflict between individual and collective needs in fair and humane ways.

Americans must also resolve the ethical dilemmas posed by the enormous power of medical intervention. How long should physical life be prolonged? Can we live with the possibilities of human genetic engineering? How premature does a fetus have to be to be considered unviable? Should society help to cover the costs of catastrophically expensive, but potentially effective, medical procedures?

Like its history, the future of health, illness, and medical care is about all of us. We all need health care. We must take responsibility for the delivery system we create. Like residents of other counties throughout the nation, McLean County citizens must examine their past and present in order to select things of value to take into the future.

Appendix

Oral History Interviews

The following people were interviewed specifically for the *A Matter of Life and Death: Health, Illness and Medicine in McLean County* project by project volunteers between April 1994 and September 1995.

NAME	YEAR OF BIRTH	RESIDENCE	OCCUPATION
Grace Allman	1896	Stanford	Teacher
Marie Bostic	1897	Danvers	Teacher
Loren Boon	1917	Washburn Danvers	Doctor (GP)
Ben Boyd	1927	Bloomington	Sanitarian
Ruth Carpenter	1909	Vermilion Co./ Bloomington/ Shirley	Nurse
Ethel Cherry	1911	Arrowsmith	Postmaster
W.L. Dillman	1920	Bloomington	Dentist
Margaret Esposito	1923	Bloomington	Home Advisor, CES
Martha Ferguson	1916	Lexington	Factory work (GE)
Richard & Mary Finfgeld	1906 (Mr.) ? (Mrs.)	Lexington	Newspaper work/ Trained Teacher/ Housewife
Roberta Holman	1921	Danvers	Nurse
Ferne Hensley	1894	Arrowsmith	Housewife
Sister Judith	1922	Düsseldorf, Germany	Nursing nun
Evelyn Lantz	1918	Danvers/ Bloomington	Nurse
Russel Oyer	1920	Bloomington	Physician (GP)
Harriet Rust	? (c. 1920)	Bloomington	?
Harold Shinall	1909	Gibson City/Bloomington	Physician (GP, Radiologist)
Marie Snyder	1899	Bloomington	Hairdresser, Housewife
Alice Swift	1927	Bloomington	Nurse
Ralph Spencer	1914	Danvers	Farmer, Mechanic, Retail
Jane Tinsley	1924	Bloomington	Nurse
Paul Theobald	1922	Bloomington	Physician (GP)
Sr. Theonilla	1912	Dortmund, Germany	Nursing nun
Albert VanNess	1926	Bloomington	Internist
Caribel Washington	1914	Bloomington	Community work/ State Farm
Sally Wagner	1938	Bloomington	Nurse
James Welch	1915	Cuba, IL	Physician (GP)
Reginald Whitaker	1925	Normal	Maintenance, GTE

The following people were interviewed by Cynthia Baer for a class project at Illinois State University during the 1992/3 academic year. Transcripts were used with Ms. Baer's permission.

Mrs. Rittenhouse	1941	Eureka	Homemaker
Mrs. Rohm	1966	Eureka	Homemaker
Mrs. Rueger	1913	Cruger	Homemaker

The following people were interviewed for the Bloomington-Normal Black History Project. Partial transcripts and notes were consulted by the author with permission.

Lucinda Brent Posey	1914	Streator/Normal
Marguerite Jackson	1927	Bloomington
Matilda Calico	1909 or 1910	Bloomington
Katherine Dean	1910	Bloomington
Dorothy Jean Stewart	1933	Bloomington
Ruth Waddell	1923	Bloomington
Oscar Waddell	1917	Bloomington
Josephine Samuels	1922	Normal
Lavada Hunter	1913	Bloomington

Notes

Introduction

[1] Of course, this area was not "discovered" by these migrants, but had indeed been inhabited by Native Americans of various tribes for centuries. These peoples had their own ways of managing ill-health, which deserve consideration in their own right and are beyond the scope of this study.

[2] Heroic therapeutic techniques are particularly associated with allopathy, which is the name given to the dominant school of professional medical practitioners. Allopaths formed the American Medical Association in 1847 and led all efforts to professionalize and regulate medical practice. However, other categories of practitioners, such as homeopaths, Thomsonians, osteopaths and eclectics won loyal supporters and defeated the allopaths' nineteenth-century attempts to obtain a legal monopoly over medical practice, partly because of patients' distaste for heroic medicine.

[3] The 1850 Census for Bloomington lists 16 men identifying themselves as "Doctors."

[4] Compare the 1839 "Day Book" of Thomas Rogers with the "Records of the McLean County Medical Society" (1891-1910), which list fee bills agreed upon by the members. Both documents are housed by the McLean County Historical Society .

[5] The exceptions to this rule were dentistry, which was conducted in offices, pharmacy, which usually took place in shops; and the occasional visits made by patients or their families to the physician's home or office — often simply to pick up a bottle of medicine. Acute or serious illness was invariably treated in the sufferer's home.

[6] I am indebted to Paul Starr's *The Social Transformation of American Medicine* New York: Basic Books (1982) for the concept of cultural authority invested in medical practitioners.

[7] Hospitals in small communities tended to be facilities owned and operated by one doctor. Dr. Johnson's Hospital in Arrowsmith, opened in the 1920s, was typical of this type of institution, as was the residential facility organized to house clients taking the Willowbark Cure in Danvers in 1892. Similar facilities were organized in larger cities, of course. The Kelso Sanitarium in Bloomington was opened primarily to treat the patients of homeopathic physicians George and Annie Kelso. Its building was sold to the Mennonite Hospital Association in 1920.

[8] See e.g., Rosemary Stevens, *In Sickness and in Wealth: American Hospitals in the Twentieth Century*, New York: Basic Books (1989), p. 172.

[9] Blue Cross, largest of the nonprofit hospital insurance (or prepayment) programs, was established in the 1930s. See Stevens, op.cit., pp. 182ff.

[10] "Records of the McLean County Medical Society," July 1, 1897, unpublished ms., McLean County Historical Society. The Society also houses a number of photographs of "classes" of goiter patients operated on by Drs. Hart and Hawks of Brokaw Hospital.

[11] This was particularly true for Brokaw Hospital, founded in 1896, whose training school was established in 1902; and Mennonite Hospital, which opened in 1919 and began training nurses in 1920. St. Joseph's Hospital, established in

1880, maintained a nurse training school between 1921 and 1962, but was dependent on its permanent "staff" of nursing nuns for most day-to-day activities.

12 The relationships between Illinois State Normal University and Brokaw Hospital's nurse training program and Mennonite Hospital's nurse training school and Illinois Wesleyan University are local examples of this trend.

13 Particular thanks are due, here, to the Order of the Sisters of St. Francis, Mennonite College of Nursing and BroMenn Health Care for opening their archives to project researchers.

1. Early Days: Suffering in McLean County

1 James H. Cassedy, *Medicine in America: A Short History*, Baltimore, MD: Johns Hopkins University Press (1991), p. 72.

2 See, e.g., Charles Rosenburg, *The Cholera Years*, Chicago: University of Chicago Press (1962), pp. 76-7.

3 Cassedy, op.cit., p. 46.

4 See, e.g., Sheila M. Rothman, *Living in the Shadow of Death: Tuberculosis and the Social Experience of Illness in American History,* Baltimore, MD: Johns Hopkins University Press (1995).

5 See Isaac D. Rawlings, *The Rise and Fall of Disease in Illinois*, Springfield, IL: Schnepp & Barnes (1927; reprinted 1994) Vol. 1, pp. 70ff. for a useful discussion of the history of the identification of typhoid as a disease separate from typhus and malaria.

6 See, e.g., George Rosen, *Preventive Medicine in the United States, 1900-1975*, New York: Science History Publications (1975), p. 4.

7 See, e.g., William McNeill, *Plagues and Peoples*, Garden City, N.Y.: Anchor Press (1976).

8 Quoted in Rawlings, op.cit., Vol. 1, p. 31.

9 Quoted in Lucius H. Zeuch, *History of Medical Practice in Illinois*, Vol. 1, Chicago: The Book Press (1927), p. 470.

10 E. Duis, *Good Old Times in McLean County*, Bloomington, IL.: The Leader Publishing and Printing House (1874), pp. 10-11.

11 Rawlings, op.cit., p. 36. See also James H. Cassedy, "Why Self Help? Americans Alone with their Diseases 1800-1850" in G. B. Risse, R. L. Numbers and J. Walzer Leavitt (eds), *Medicine Without Doctors: Home Health Care in American History*, New York: Science History Publications (1977), p. 42.

12 Daniel Drake, *A Systematic Treatise Historical, Etiological, and Practical on the Principal Diseases of the Interior Valley of North America*, Vol. 2, New York: Burt Franklin (1971 reprint: first published 1854), p. 56.

13 Marlin Ray Ingalls, "The Espy Pharmacy Records," unpublished Illinois State University Master's thesis (1986), p. 14.

14 Rawlings, op.cit., Vol. 2, p. 57.

15 ibid., pp. 45, 320-27.

16 ibid., p. 44.

17 Ingalls, op.cit., p. 15, refers to an 1882 *Pantagraph* report on Bloomington's treatment of foreigners and travelers from epidemic areas. These people were "scrutinized outside of town or not allowed to disembark within the city limits."

18 ibid., p. 70.

19 Judith Walzer Leavitt, *Brought to Bed: Childbearing in America*, 1750-1950, New York: Oxford University Press (1986), pp. 24-5.

[20] Rawlings, op.cit., Vol. 1, p.85.

[21] ibid., p. 394. There are accurate records for neither deaths nor causes of death for earlier years.

[22] ibid., p. 87.

[23] Drake, op.cit., pp. 520-1.

[24] Data included in this table were extracted from Isaac D. Rawlings, *The Rise and Fall of Disease in Illinois*, Springfield, IL.: Schnepp & Barnes (1927; reprinted 1994), pp. 311-88.

[25] See e.g., Emily K. Abel, "Family Caregiving in the Nineteenth Century: Emily Hawley Gillespie and Sarah Gillespie, 1858-1888," *Bulletin of the History of Medicine*, vol. 68, no. 4, pp. 573-99.

[26] J.B. Orendorff, "Sketch of Major Baker," unpublished ms., McLean County Historical Society .

[27] Morris Fishbein (ed), *Modern Home Medical Adviser*, New York: Doubleday, Doran (1935), Preface.

[28] *The Home Cook Book of Chicago*, Chicago: J. Fred. Waggoner (1874), p. 267.

[29] John B. Blake, "From Buchan to Fishbein: The Literature of Domestic Medicine" in *Medicine Without Doctors*, op.cit., pp. 11-30.

[30] Quoted in ibid., p. 20.

[31] The McLean County Historical Society contains a number of prescriptions, written in the form of recipes which could be compounded by either sufferer or pharmacist.

[32] J.B. Orendorff, "Sketch of Omen and Zena Olney," unpublished ms., McLean County Historical Society . The mixture referred to was probably red precipitate, or red oxide of mercury, which is both water soluble and poisonous.

[33] Beatrice Armstrong, "Silas Hubbard, Early Physician of McLean County," unpublished ms., McLean County Historical Society.

[34] Quoted in Blake, op.cit., p. 18.

[35] Duis, op.cit., p. 541.

[36] J.B. Orendorff, "Sketch of Omen and Zena Olney," op.cit., p. 7.

[37] Espy is mentioned in neither the several catalogues of biographies of local worthies in early county histories, nor in the *Biographical History* published by the McLean County Medical Society. Thus, no information about his credentials is available. However, it seems likely that he was related to John E. Espy who ran a drug store in Bloomington between 1873 and 1884.

[38] J.B. Orendorff, "Sketch of Major Baker," op.cit., p. 3.

[39] J.B. Orendorff, "Sketch of Omen and Zena Olney," op.cit., p. 3.

[40] Duis, op.cit., p. 297.

[41] This having been said, there is a long history of women using herbal, mechanical, magical and other means to prevent pregnancy or procure abortion. Traditionally, such matters were only legally regulated if managed by "professionals"; self treatment was regarded as the woman's own business by secular society. Abortion was traditionally regarded as acceptable before "quickening" (the point in her pregnancy when the mother felt her baby move).

[42] Leavitt, op.cit., pp. 28-32.

[43] ibid., pp. 14, 19.

2. Healing in McLean County: Doctors and Doctoring in the Nineteenth Century

1 James H. Cassedy, *Medicine in America: A Short History*, Baltimore, MD: Johns Hopkins University Press (1991), p. 41.

2 Paul Starr, *The Social Transformation of American Medicine*, New York: Basic Books (1982), p. 104.

3 Cassedy, op.cit., pp. 89-90.

4 See Norman Gevitz, *Other Healers: Unorthodox Medicine in America*, Baltimore, MD: Johns Hopkins University Press (1988).

5 ibid., p. 38. See also Martin Kaufman, *Homeopathy in America: The Rise and Fall of a Medical Heresy*, Baltimore, MD: Johns Hopkins University Press (1971).

6 Not included here are discussions of theories tangentially related to medicine, such as phrenology, which profiled human character, potential and behavior according to skull shape, and mesmerism, which employed hypnosis to cure and entertain. The nineteenth century also gave birth to psychology, which developed a secular scientific basis for the study of human thought processes and the treatment of emotional illnesses. In addition, various religious sects, notably Christian Science, encouraged adherents to deal with health problems by spiritual means.

7 See Norman Gevitz, *The D.O.s: Osteopathic Medicine in America*, Baltimore, MD: Johns Hopkins University Press (1982).

8 Cassedy, op.cit., p. 100.

9 This pattern of nostrum concoction and marketing had been quite traditional in early modern Europe, and presaged the development of the patent medicine market. Many otherwise respectable practitioners sold their own "secret" remedies which promised to cure everything from vague malaise to cancers. Thus, nineteenth-century quacks shared a long history with regular physicians and surgeons.

10 Wakefield, born in 1815, had been a farmer and schoolteacher before joining his brother Zera, who was actually a physician, in the nostrum trade. After Zera's death, the business became extraordinarily successful, making Dr. Cyrenius Wakefield a wealthy and powerful man. See, e.g., Jacob L. Hasbrouck, *History of McLean County Illinois*, Topeka-Indianapolis: Historical Publishing Company (1924), pp. 408ff.

11 ibid., p. 267.

12 Bateman, Newton (ed.), *Historical Encyclopedia of Illinois and History of McLean County*, Chicago: Munsell Publishing Co. (1908), Vol. 2, p. 850.

13 Cassedy, op.cit., p. 32

14 ibid.

15 ibid., p. 27.

16 ibid.

17 At approximately one physician for every 100 people, the doctor/patient ratio compares extremely favorably to both the current U.S. government desirable ratio of one primary care physician per 3,500 population and the state of Illinois' standard of one primary care physician per 2,400.

18 See the previous chapter for a discussion of Drake's study of diseases in the Midwest.

19 E. Duis, *Good Old Times in McLean County*, Bloomington, IL.: The Leader Publishing and Printing House (1874), pp. 261-2.

20 *The History of McLean County, Illinois*, Chicago: Wm. Le Baron, Jr., & Co. (1879), p. 773.

21 Thomas P. Rogers, "Day Books" (April 1839-September, 1841; January, 1850-April,1854), unpublished ms., McLean County Historical Society.

22 Local sources do not provide the name of the medical school Rogers attended — a fact which is both unusual and suspicious, particularly since Rogers became very active in state business and politics, hobnobbing with worthies such as Stephen Douglas and Abraham Lincoln.

23 Duis, op.cit., pp. 846-852.

24 Hasbrouck, op.cit., p. 267.

25 Bateman, op.cit., p. 851.

26 See Michael G. Matejka and Greg Koos, *Bloomington's C. & A. Shops: Our Lives Remembered*, Bloomington, IL: McLean County Historical Society (1987).

27 Cassedy, op.cit., p. 26. By 1870, there were more than 400 medical societies in the United States, formed by allopaths to improve the standards of medical practice and to keep alternative practitioners and quacks from establishing themselves locally.

28 These take the form of a reprint of the original constitution and brief biographies of early members contained in the *Biographical History of the Members of the McLean County Medical Society and Other Physicians Who Have Practiced Medicine in McLean County, 1854-1934,* published by the McLean County Medical Society in 1934.

29 "Records of the McLean County Medical Society, 1891-1910," unpublished ms., McLean County Historical Society.

30 *Biographical History*, op.cit., p. 8.

31 All references to Society activities for the years between 1891 and 1910 have as their source the *Records of the McLean County Medical Society*, op.cit., unless otherwise indicated.

32 *Biographical History*, op.cit., p. 74.

33 Starr, op.cit., p. 69.

34 "Records," 3/9/07.

35 See, e.g., "Records," 6/4/1894, 12/2/1897, 6/6/01.

36 "Records," 11/3/04.

37 Bateman, op.cit., p. 852.

38 Hasbrouck, op.cit., Vol. 2, p. 1089.

39 ibid.

3. Cleanliness Is Next to Godliness: Public Health and Personal Hygiene

1 Isaac D. Rawlings, *The Rise and Fall of Disease in Illinois*, Springfield, IL.: Schnepp & Barnes (1927; reprinted 1994), Vol. 1, p. 410.

2 *Profile of Illinois' Elderly*, Springfield, IL: Illinois Department on Aging (1994), p.1.

3 See, e.g., Andrew Boorde, *The Breviary of Health,* London (1587).

4 See, e.g., *The Diary of Samuel Pepys*, R. Latham and W. Matthews, (eds), vols I-IX, Berkeley: University of California Press (1970-82). The seventeenth-century English diarist had suffered greatly from bladder stones, which were surgically removed. Thereafter, Pepys devoted a good deal of time to planning and trying to follow rules of good health, which largely consisted of eating sensibly and not

becoming constipated. See also Lucinda McCray Beier, *Sufferers and Healers: The Experience of Illness in Seventeenth-Century England*, London: Routledge and Kegan Paul (1987) for a general discussion of diarists' methods of preventing and dealing with illness.

5 See, e.g., Charles Rosenburg, *The Cholera Years*, Chicago: University of Chicago Press (1962).

6 Catharine E. Beecher, *Letters to the People on Health and Happiness*, New York: Arno Press and the New York Times (1972 reprint of the 1855 edition), p. 71. Beecher's thoughts are heavily drawn upon here, partly because she taught Sarah Davis, and thus is known to have had some local influence. Beecher also represents the progressive spectrum of health advocates of the time, having a particular interest in the health of women.

7 Perhaps more than any century except our own, the 1800s gave rise to a huge range of theories about healthy eating habits. The prescribed composition of diets and appropriate ways of consuming food differed enormously from one expert to another. Indeed, the health fads of the nineteenth century stimulated the development of certain foods which have become dietary staples in this century (notably graham crackers and cold breakfast cereals).

8 Beecher, op.cit., pp. 62-3.

9 ibid., p. 78.

10 ibid., pp. 150, 154.

11 Quoted in Kevin W. Avery's unpublished paper "Privial Pursuit: A Research Paper on Outhouses" (1985), McLean County Historical Society.

12 Avery, op.cit., p. 4.

13 Quoted in Marlin Ray Ingalls, "The Espy Pharmacy Records," unpublished Master's thesis, Illinois State University (1986), p. 8.

14 David A. Walitschek, "Historic Archaeological Investigations at the Reuben Benjamin House," unpublished Master's thesis, Illinois State University (1988), p. 30.

15 Clover Lawn's grandness reflected the status of its owners. David Davis (1815-1886) was a Bloomington-based lawyer, judge and politician whose friendship with Abraham Lincoln won him a Supreme Court appointment in 1862. After his resignation from the Supreme Court in 1876, Davis served a six-year term in the U.S. Senate. Sarah Davis (1814-1879) was born into a prosperous Massachusetts family and was educated at the Hartford Female Seminary, where Catharine and Harriet Beecher taught. She married David Davis in 1838 and moved to Bloomington, where Davis had recently purchased Jesse Fell's law practice. Since Judge Davis's career forced him to spend much time away from home, Sarah Davis ran the household independently and made many decisions about the construction of Clover Lawn.

16 Walitschek, op.cit., p.30..

17 Rawlings, *Rise and Fall*, Vol. 2, p. 57.

18 Ingalls, op.cit., p.10.

19 ibid., p. 9. Vaccination occurred despite strong local anti-vaccination feeling.

20 ibid.

21 Rawlings, *Rise and Fall*, Vol. 2, pp. 57-9.

22 "Records of the McLean County Medical Society," unpublished ms., McLean County Historical Society.

23 Rawlings, op.cit., Vol. 2, p. 59.

24 Walitschek, op.cit., p. 29.

25 ibid., p. 30.

26 *The History of McLean County, Illinois*, Chicago: Wm. Le Baron, Jr., & Co. (1879), p. 387.

27 ibid., p. 388.

28 ibid.

29 Ingalls, op.cit., p. 8.

30 Rawlings, op.cit., vol. 2, p. 53.

31 ibid., pp. 55-6.

32 *The Pantagraph*, 4/14/68 and 1971 (McLean County Historical Society clipping file.)

33 Ingalls, op.cit., p. 6.

34 ibid., p. 7.

35 Rawlings, op.cit., p. 56.

36 ibid, p. 53.

37 *The Pantagraph*, 7/13/25, 10/2/25. J.L. Hasbrouck, *Bloomington and Normal Sanitary District, 1919-1936*, privately published (1936), pp. 5-9.

38 Rawlings, op.cit., Vol. 1, p. 131.

39 Ingalls, op.cit., p. 5.

40 Rawlings, op.cit., Vol. 2, p. 50.

41 See, e.g., Paul Starr, *The Social Transformation of American Medicine*, New York: Basic Books (1982), pp. 180-97.

42 "Records of the McLean County Medical Society", unpublished ms., McLean County Historical Society.

43 Rawlings, op.cit., Vol. 2, p. 51.

44 Margaret Esposito, *Places of Pride: The Work and Photography of Clara R. Brian*, Bloomington, IL: McLean County Historical Society (1989).

45 Oral history transcript, McLean County Historical Society, Mr. B3MP, p. 42. For reference purposes, oral history interviewees have been assigned codes.

46 Rawlings, op.cit., Vol. 2, p. 60.

47 Peoria passed such an ordinance in 1906. See, ibid., Vol. 1, p. 368.

48 ibid.

49 "Records of the McLean County Medical Society," op.cit.

50 J.L. Hasbrouck, *History of McLean County Illinois*, Topeka-Indianapolis: Historical Publishing Company (1924), Vol. 1, p. 333.

51 According to H. Clay Tate, *The Way it was in McLean County, 1972-1822*, Bloomington, IL: McLean County History '72 Association (1972), p. 254, there were only four patients in the sanitarium at this time, and 1,000 empty tuberculosis beds in the state.

52 See, e.g., Daniel M. Fox, *Power and Illness: The Failure and Future of American Health Policy*, Berkeley: University of California Press (1993).

4. Health in a Bottle: Patent Medicines and Self-Treatment

1 A. Walker Bingham, *The Snake-Oil Syndrome: Patent Medicine Advertising*, Hanover, MA: The Christopher Publishing House (1994), p. 3.

2 James Harvey Young, "Patent Medicines and the Self-Help Syndrome," in Risse, Numbers and Leavitt (eds), *Medicine Without Doctors: Home Health Care in American History*, New York: Science History Publications (1977), p. 95.

3 Bingham, op.cit., p. 5.

4 See, e.g., Lucinda McCray Beier, *Sufferers and Healers: The Experience of Illness in Seventeenth-Century England*, London: Routledge and Kegan Paul (1987), pp. 21-2.

5 ibid., pp. 14-15.

6 James H. Cassedy, *Medicine in America: A Short History*, Baltimore, MD: Johns Hopkins University Press (1991), p. 60.

7 Young, "Patent Medicines and Self Help," op.cit., p. 98.

8 Indeed, snake oil was apparently actually used as a medical ingredient. Clark Stanely's Snake Oil Liniment was marketed by a Rhode Island Drug Company during the mid-nineteenth century. See Bingham, op.cit., p. 17.

9 *The Pantagraph*, 1884. Reference appears in Marlin Ray Ingalls, "The Espy Pharmacy Records," unpublished Master's thesis, Illinois State University (1986), p. 65.

10 ibid.

11 Advertised in the *Weekly National Flag* (November 28, 1856): "For sale in Bloomington by Waters & Richardson, Crothers & Chew, Wakefield & Thompson and Paist & Marmon."

12 R.L. Oyer, M.D., "Of Doctors and Sickness in Chenoa: A Historical Perspective," unpublished ms. prepared for the Chenoa Historical Society (1992), p. 7.

13 "Day Books" of Dr. Thomas P. Rogers, unpublished ms., McLean County Historical Society.

14 *The History of McLean County, Illinois*, Chicago: Wm. Le Baron Jr., & Co. (1879), pp. 1073-77.

15 Bingham, *Snake-Oil Syndrome*, p. 6. This term was also used for remedies compounded by the druggist according to a doctor's prescription.

16 Ingalls, "Espy Pharmacy Records," p. 69.

17 Ilyse D. Barkan, "Industry Invites Regulation: The Passage of the Pure Food and Drug Act of 1906," *American Journal of Public Health*, vol. 75, no. 1 (1985), p. 22.

18 *Weekly National Flag*, Bloomington, Illinois (1850s): McLean County Historical Society.

19 ibid., [date uncertain: 1856-9 printed on back of photocopy.]

20 ibid.

21 *The People's Home Journal*, New York: F.M. Lupton. The bound volume for 1900 boasts that a total of 4,860,000 copies of this monthly magazine were sold that year.

22 Ingalls, op.cit., p. 65.

23 ibid., p. 64.

24 *The Wanamaker Diary*, Philadelphia, New York and Paris (1910), p. 55.

25 *Weekly National Flag*, loc.cit.

26 Judith Walzer Leavitt, *Brought to Bed: Childbearing in America, 1750-1950*, New York: Oxford University Press (1986), pp. 29-30.

27 The ovariotomy conducted by the Kentucky physician Ephraim McDowell in 1809 on a kitchen table without benefit of anesthetic must certainly be considered in this category.

28 See, e.g., Regina Morantz, "The Lady and Her Physician" in Mary Hartman and Lois W. Banner (eds), *Clio's Consciousness Raised: New Perspectives on the History of Women*, New York: Harper & Row (1974), pp. 38-53; and Sarah Stage, *Female Complaints: Lydia Pinkham and the Business of Women's Medicine*, New York: W. W. Norton & Co. (1979), pp. 79-82.

29 "Records of the McLean County Medical Society, 1891-1910," unpublished ms., McLean County Historical Society.

[30] *Weekly National Flag*, [1856-9].

[31] ibid.

[32] See Stage, op.cit., for a thorough treatment of Pinkham's biography and the historical contexts within which the marketing and distribution of her Vegetable Compound flourished.

[33] Young, "Patent Medicines and Self Help," op.cit., p. 103.

[34] Stage, op.cit., p. 146.

[35] ibid., p. 147.

[36] ibid.

[37] ibid., pp. 155-6.

[38] Advertising flier, McLean County Historical Society. Since Dr. Rue is not mentioned in the *Biographical History of the Members of the McLean County Medical Society*, it is possible that he was not a licensed physician but was, like Cyrenius Wakefield, a patent medicine "doctor."

[39] Jacob L. Hasbrouck, *History of McLean County Illinois*, Topeka-Indianapolis: Historical Publishing Company (1924), Vol. 1, p. 409. See also. E. Duis, *Good Old Times in McLean County*, Bloomington, IL: The Leader Publisher and Printing (1874), pp. 354-8 and Linda Kay Plummer, "Medicine Factory" in *Illinois History*, vol. 16, no. 1 (1962), p. 10.

[40] "An Autobiography of Dr. Cyrenius Wakefield," revised by Dr. Homer Wakefield, Bloomington, IL: (1889?), unpublished ms., McLean County Historical Society.

[41] Duis, op.cit., p. 357.

[42] Ingalls, op.cit., pp. 126-7.

[43] McLean County Historical Society.

[44] Ironically, many of his trips to places like Florida, California and Colorado Springs were apparently taken for his health or that of family members. See entries for 1880 and 1883, "An Autobiography of Dr. Cyrenius Wakefield," op.cit.

[45] Hasbrouck, op.cit., Vol. 1, p. 409.

[46] James Harvey Young, *The Medical Messiahs: A Social History of Health Quackery in Twentieth-Century America*, Princeton, N.J.: Princeton University Press (1967), p. 23.

[47] Ingalls, op.cit., pp. 67-8.

[48] The Anchor Electric Belt was advertised in *Good Literature*, New York: F.M. Lupton, January 1900.

[49] Barkan, "Industry Invites Regulation," *American Journal of Public Health*, vol. 75, no. 1, (1985), p. 22.

[50] Quoted in Young, *Medical Messiahs*, op.cit., p. 31.

[51] ibid., p. 23.

[52] ibid., pp. 36-7.

5. Away From Home: Hospital Development

[1] From very early days, European lepers had been confined in lazar houses. After the advent of syphilis in late fifteenth-century Europe, sufferers too poor to be cared for at home sometimes were hospitalized; St. Thomas's Hospital in London specialized in treatment of the "French Pox." Beginning in the early modern period, the emotionally ill were also increasingly confined in hospitals.

[2] There were always a small number of high-status physicians with hospital appointments. For example, William Harvey had an appointment at St. Bartholomew's Hospital, London, in the early seventeenth century. The value of and interest in these appointments expanded after urban hospitals began to be strongly associated with research and teaching in the late eighteenth century.

[3] James H. Cassedy, *Medicine in America*, Baltimore, MD: Johns Hopkins University Press (1991) , p. 19.

[4] Rosemary Stevens, *In Sickness and in Wealth: American Hospitals in the Twentieth Century*, New York: Basic Books (1989), p. 20.

[5] Charles E. Rosenberg, *The Care of Strangers; The Rise of America's Hospital System*, New York: Basic Books (1987), p. 5.

[6] ibid.

[7] Stevens, op.cit., p. 9.

[8] Rosenberg, op.cit., pp. 4, 5, 122. Paul Starr, *The Social Transformation of American Medicine*, New York: Basic Books ((1982), p. 157.

[9] Stevens, op.cit., p. 20.

[10] ibid.

[11] Starr, op.cit.

[12] Rosenberg, op.cit., p. 111.

[13] Stevens, op.cit., p. 25.

[14] Rosenberg, op.cit., pp. 43-4.

[15] So useful and cost effective were student nurses that even Catholic hospitals staffed by professional nursing Sisters often opened nurse training schools. St. Joseph's Hospital (Bloomington) operated such a school between 1921 and 1962.

[16] The history of nursing is more fully discussed in Chapter 6.

[17] Stevens, op.cit., p. 173.

[18] Starr, op.cit., p. 359.

[19] ibid., pp. 178-9.

[20] ibid., p. 29.

[21] Corlin Ferguson, "The McLean County Poor Farm," unpublished report produced for the "A Matter of Life and Death: Health, Illness and Medicine in McLean County" project, p. 3, McLean County Historical Society. When the state assumed responsibility for institutional care of the insane, the County decided not to build an asylum. However, both local charitable hospitals and the Poor Farm continued to house the emotionally ill well into the twentieth century.

[22] ibid., p. 5.

[23] ibid., p. 10.

[24] This development was also fairly typical of Illinois counties; by 1948, 23 counties had converted their poor farms into nursing homes.

[25] *The Pantagraph*, 3/22/1892.

[26] Stevens, op.cit., p. 29. St. Joseph's Hospital will be dealt with at greater length following chapter 5 in a case study of the hospital's operation, 1880-1910.

[27] Two Sisters of German origin participated in oral history interviews for this project. One emigrated during the 1930s, while the other emigrated in the early 1950s.

[28] Jacob L. Hasbrouck, *History of McLean County Illinois*, Topeka-Indianapolis: Historical Publishing Company (1924), Vol. 2, pp. 1088-9.

[29] It is noteworthy that their names do not appear in the 1904 list of members printed in the *Biographical History of the Members of the McLean County Medical Society*. While George Kelso appears on the 1934 list, Annie is mentioned only as his wife, despite the fact that both had medical degrees from the

University of Michigan.

[30] Marketing brochure for the "Kelso Sanitarium." Although this document is undated, it was probably produced in 1916, since "the dedication of our new building," accomplished in that year according to Jacob Hasbrouck (op.cit., Vol. 2, p. 1089), is mentioned on page 3.

[31] "Kelso Sanitarium," p. 4.

[32] Mrs. R4MP, p.3

[33] In 1928, Brokaw Hospital was charging $4.00 per day.

[34] 1897 letter from the Rev. J.A. Springer of the Society of Light and Hope (Chicago), quoted in Maude F. Essig's unpublished essay, "History of Brokaw Hospital" (1939), p. 3, Mennonite College of Nursing Library.

[35] ibid., p. 4.

[36] Steven R. Estes, *Christian Concern for Health: The Sixtieth Anniversary History of the Mennonite Hospital Association*, Bloomington, IL: The Assocaition (1979), p. 12.

[37] Mr. F2MP, p. 25.

[38] Mrs. H2MP, p. 5; *Biographical History of the Members of the McLean County Medical Society, 1854-1934*, McLean County Medical Society (1934), p. 59.

[39] Estes, op.cit., p. 101.

[40] This development was similar to the founding of the Keeley Institute in Dwight, Illinois, in 1879 by Leslie E. Keeley, a railroad surgeon. This Institute operated until 1966. The Keeley Gold Cure was available, either at the Institute or by mail order. See A. Walker Bingham, *The Snake-Oil Syndrome: Patent Medicine Advertising*, Hanover, MA: The Christopher Publishing House (1994), pp. 44-5.

[41] *Danvers, Illinois Community History*, Danvers Historical Society, Inc. (1987), pp. 48-9; Corlin R. Ferguson, "Willow Bark Institute," unpublished paper, McLean County Historical Society.

[42] *The Pantagraph*, 8/28/1994.

[43] Estes, op.cit., p. 43.

[44] ibid., p. 62.

[45] ibid., pp. 64, 65, 87.

[46] Essig, op.cit., p. 12.

[47] "Brokaw Hospital Annual Report," 1930.

[48] "St. Joseph's Hospital Accounts, 1880-97, " Archives of The Sisters of the Third Order of St. Francis, Peoria, Illinois. In Spring, 1882, the Sisters sold "chances on a watch" — a fairly lucrative effort which raised over $100 in a three-month period. In July, 1888, there is reference to the sale of raffle tickets.

[49] Essig, op.cit., p. 3.

[50] Estes, op.cit., p. 20.

[51] ibid., p. 18.

[52] A. Edward Livingston, *A History of the Practice of Medicine in McLean County, Illinois 1930-1980*, privately published (1989), p. 3; Estes, op.cit., p. 48.

[53] Estes, op.cit., p. 49.

[54] ibid., p. 92; Stevens, *In Sickness and in Wealth*, p. 201; information about St. Joseph's and Brokaw's receipt of this funding was provided by the hospitals themselves.

[55] Stevens, op.cit., p. 172

[56] ibid., 182.

[57] Brokaw Hospital, 1920 promotional pamphlet. The figure of nine surgeons is actually an underestimate, since the four Eye, Ear, Nose and Throat specialists

and the Gynecologist also did a great deal of surgery.

58 Estes, op.cit., p. 47.

59 ibid., pp. 22, 50, 61, 64.

60 "Kelso Sanitarium," pp. 12-14; Estes, op.cit., p. 49.

61 "St. Joseph's Hospital Accounts," op.cit.

62 Mrs. R4MP, p. 4.

63 Essig, op.cit., pp. 24-5.

64 Estes, op.cit., p. 97.

65 Essig, op.cit., p. 10.

66 Brokaw Hospital, 1920 promotional pamphlet, p. 12.

67 R. W. and D. C. Wertz, *Lying-In: A History of Childbirth in America*, New York: The Free Press (1977), p. 133.

68 Estes, op.cit., p. 95.

69 This study is indebted to Preston Hawks for his exhaustive research on polio in McLean County.

70 *Danvers, Illinois Community History*, op.cit., p. 48.

Case Study: St. Joseph's Hospital, 1880-1906

1 Biographical information about early St. Joseph's staff members appears in the *Biographical History of the Members of the McLean County Medical Society, 1854-1934*, (1934).

2 "St. Joseph's Medical Staff Records," pp. 16, 34, Archives of The Sisters of the Third Order of St. Francis, Peoria, Illinois.

3 ibid., p. 16.

4 ibid., 1886, p. 12.

5 ibid., pp. 8-9.

6 ibid., pp. 11, 23.

7 ibid., p. 25.

8 ibid., pp. 36, 24, 45.

9 ibid., p. 38.

10 ibid., pp. 38, 40; "St. Joseph's Hospital Accounts," p. 257, Archives of The Sisters of the Third Order of St. Francis, Peoria, Illinois.

11 "St. Joseph's Medical Staff Records," p. 30, Archives of The Sisters of the Third Order of St. Francis, Peoria, Illinois..

12 ibid., p. 47.

13 ibid., p. 17.

14 ibid., p. 13; *St. Joseph's Hospital Admissions Records*, 1880-1906.

15 "St. Joseph's Medical Staff Records," p. 47.

16 For discussion of the Poor Farm's consideration of this issue, see Corlin R. Ferguson, "The McLean County Poor Farm," unpublished ms., McLean County Historical Society.

17 "St. Joseph's Hospital Admissions Records."

18 "St. Joseph's Medical Staff Records," p. 55. These rooms were apparently still in use during the mid-twentieth century, according to oral history respondents.

19 Charles Rosenberg, *The Care of Strangers*, New York: Basic Books (1987), p. 111.

20 Race was not always noted in the "Admissions Records." Sometimes race was recorded for both black and white patients; sometimes it is indicated only for

black patients.

[21] In 1916 the County was paying $1 per day to local hospitals for the care of the indigent. See Corlin Ferguson, op.cit.

[22] "St. Joseph's Medical Staff Records," p. 34.

[23] "St. Joseph's Hospital Accounts."

[24] Included in the category of miscellaneous illnesses are acute exyemia, anaemia, brain trouble, chronic eczema, congestion of brain, general debility, granulated eyelids, jaundice, liver complaint, metritis, old age, palsy, papilonia, paralysis, shingles, hives, sore eye, spinal clinosis, tapeworms, and torpid liver.

[25] "St. Joseph's Medical Staff Records," p. 29.

[26] ibid., p. 28.

[27] ibid., p. 39.

[28] ibid., p. 17.

[29] "St. Joseph's Hospital Accounts," pp. 26, 56, 146.

[30] "St. Joseph's Medical Staff Records," p. 28.

[31] "St. Joseph's Hospital Accounts," pp. 130, 132.

[32] "St. Joseph's Medical Staff Records," p. 16.

6. Caring For Strangers: Nurse Training and Nursing

[1] Susan M. Reverby, *Ordered to Care: The Dilemma of American Nursing, 1850-1945*, New York: Cambridge University Press (1987), p. 47ff.

[2] Quoted in ibid., p. 54.

[3] ibid., p. 63.

[4] Reprinted by The Sisters of the Third Order of St. Francis for St. John's Hospital commemorating their one hundred years of service in Springfield, Illinois: Archives of the Third Order of the Sisters of St. Francis, Peoria, Illinois.

[5] Reverby, op.cit., pp. 121-3.

[6] Brian T. Gegel, "Formation and the First Fifty Years of the 6th District Illinois Nurses' Association," unpublished 1992 paper, Illinois Wesleyan University.

[7] Reverby, op.cit., p. 165.

[8] Indeed, Mennonite Hospital inherited and continued Kelso's nursing school when it purchased the Kelso Sanitarium.

[9] The exact date of the opening of Deaconess/Brokaw Hospital's nursing school is difficult to ascertain. According to Brokaw's own promotional literature, the school was established in 1902. However, Maude Essig's 1939 "History of Brokaw Hospital"(Mennonite College of Nursing Library) indicates that, "In November 1899, Miss Jefferson [the head deaconess] announced to the Board the coming graduating exercises for the student nurses. It was voted that announcement of same be made in each church with a cordial invitation for the public to attend." (p. 4) This suggests that the Methodist Deaconesses were training students from the time they arrived in Bloomington.

[10] Lori Ann Musser, "Nursing Education at Illinois Wesleyan University: 1923 to 1976," unpublished paper, Illinois Wesleyan University. Probable date, 1976.

[11] *Mennonite Hospital School of Nursing: The Passing of the Flame*, Bloomington, IL: Mennonite College of Nursing (1985), p. 64.

[12] Oral history transcripts are coded for ease of reference. Mrs. H1MP, p. 37.

[13] Mrs. H1MP, p. 16.

[14] Mrs. T1MP, p. 13.

[15] Mrs. C1MP, p. 38.

[16] Sr. J1MP, p. 4.
[17] Mrs. L1MP, p. 5.
[18] ibid., pp. 6-7.
[19] Mrs. S2MP, pp. 7, 14.
[20] Brokaw Hospital informational pamphlet, 1921, p. 17.
[21] ibid., p. 18.
[22] ibid., p17.
[23] Mrs. C1MP, pp. 38, 43.
[24] Mrs. L1MP, p. 7.
[25] Mrs. W2MP, p. 20.
[26] Mrs. C1MP, p. 39.
[27] Mrs. H1MP, p. 38.
[28] Mrs. S2MP, pp. 18-19.
[29] ibid., p. 21.
[30] Mrs. W2MP, p. 17.
[31] Mrs. L1MP, pp. 3-4.
[32] Mrs. C1MP, p. 40.
[33] ibid., p. 74.
[34] Mrs. T1MP, p. 17.
[35] Mrs. H1MP, p. 30.
[36] Mrs. C1MP, p. 49.
[37] Mrs. H1MP, p. 30.
[38] Mrs. L1MP, p. 38.
[39] Mrs. C1MP, p. 23.
[40] Mrs. W2MP, p. 26.
[41] Mrs. H1MP, p. 30.
[42] ibid., pp. 41, 46.
[43] Sr. T3MP, pp. 10, 21.
[44] Essig, "History of Brokaw Hospital," p. 17.
[45] Mrs. C1MP, p. 46.
[46] Mrs. L1MP, p. 28.
[47] Mrs. C1MP, pp. 45, 52.
[48] Mrs. W2MP, p. 18.
[49] See ibid., p. 54.
[50] Mrs. W2MP, p. 20.
[51] Mrs. T1MP, p. 17.
[52] Mrs. L1MP, pp. 22, 23, 24.
[53] Mrs. W2MP, p. 27.
[54] Mrs. S2MP, pp. 19-20.
[55] Mrs. L1MP, p. 22.
[56] Mrs. H1MP, pp. 18-19.
[57] Mrs. C1MP, p. 44.
[58] Mrs. W2MP, p. 18.
[59] "BroMenn Healthcare Historical Program - Script" (1992), p. 4.
[60] Mrs. C1MP, p. 61,
[61] Sr. T3MP, p. 26.
[62] Mrs. C1MP, p. 57-8.
[63] ibid., p. 47.
[64] ibid., p. 48
[65] ibid., pp. 75-6.
[66] ibid., p. 47.

[67] Mrs. H1MP, p. 27.

[68] BroMenn Healthcare archives.

[69] Mrs. C1MP, p. 58.

[70] Steven R. Estes, *Christian Concern for Health: The Sixtieth Anniversary History of the Mennonite Hospital Association,* Bloomington, IL: Mennonite Hospital Association (1979) p. 56.

[71] *The Pantagraph,* 5/5/46.

[72] Reverby, *Ordered to Care.,* p. 204.

[73] Mrs. T1MP, p. 26.

[74] Sr. T3MP pp. 39-40.

[75] Mrs. H1MP, p. 58.

[76] Sr. T3MP, p. 57.

[77] ibid., pp. 53-55.

[78] ibid., p. 40.

[79] Mrs. L1MP, p. 25.

[80] Mrs. S2MP, pp. 55-6.

[81] Mrs. T1MP, p. 23.

[82] Mrs. H1MP, p. 37.

[83] Mrs. W2MP, pp. 14, 27.

[84] *Liquorian,* vol. 57, no. 6 (1969)

7. To Do No Harm: Healing in The Twentieth-Century

[1] Gert H. Brieger, "Surgery in Late Nineteenth-Century America" in C. Lawrence (ed.), *Medical Theory, Surgical Practice,* London: Routledge and Kegan Paul (1992) p. 228.

[2] Isaac D. Rawlings, *The Rise and Fall of Disease in Illinois,* Vol. 1, Springfield, Illinois: Schnepp & Barnes (1927; reprinted 1994), p. 281.

[3] It is noteworthy that states continue to face the challenge of licensing graduates from schools they cannot regulate. According to Dr. A. Edward Livingston in his *A History of the Practice of Medicine in McLean County, Illinois, 1930-1980* (1989), "The Illinois State Medical Society passed a resolution asking that the state licensing board make provisions to certify Gudalajara [Autonomous University of Guadalajara, Mexico] graduates and also those from other equally adequate foreign schools so they could practice in Illinois. This was called the 'Fifth Pathway' and entailed further study in recognized teaching hospitals in the United States and the passing of certain tests. This resolution was presented to the State Legislature and was acted on favorably in 1972." (p. 16)

[4] *Annual Report of the President of Harvard College, 1869-70,* p. 18 and the *Annual Report of the President of Harvard College, 1871-72,* pp. 25-6, as quoted in Paul Starr, *The Social Transformation of American Medicine,* New York: Basic Books (1982), p. 113.

[5] ibid., p. 114.

[6] ibid., p. 115.

[7] Commercial, or proprietary, schools were run for profit. Usually without association with hospitals or universities, generally without full-time faculty members, they accepted students based upon their ability to pay the school's fees in advance. The academic year was short; four months was typical. Thus, both students and faculty members were able to work and earn during the rest of the

year.
[8] Thomas Neville Bonner, *Medicine in Chicago, 1850-1950*, Madison, WI: The American History Research Center (1957), p. 112.

[9] Starr, op.cit., pp. 117-8.

[10] ibid., p. 118.

[11] ibid., pp. 118-20.

[12] ibid., p. 121.

[13] ibid., p. 122.

[14] ibid., pp. 117, 124.

[15] Bonner, op.cit., p. 58.

[16] *Biographical History of the McLean County Medical Society, 1854-1954*, Bloomington, IL: McLean County Medical Society (1954), pp. 23, 41.

[17] ibid., pp. 23, 76.

[18] Bonner, op.cit., pp. 108-9.

[19] ibid., pp. 114, 115.

[20] ibid., p. 63.

[21] It is also enhanced by two local histories of medicine written by retired physicians. *A History of the Practice of Medicine in McLean County, Illinois 1930-1980* was written and privately published in 1989 by A. Edward Livingston, M.D., who practiced internal medicine in Bloomington between 1946 and 1985. *Of Doctors and Sickness in Chenoa — A Historical Perspective* was prepared for the Chenoa Historical Society in 1992 by Dr. Russell L. Oyer, who was a general practitioner in Chenoa between 1954 until his retirement in 1990.

[22] Dr. D1MP, pp. 7-8.

[23] *Biographical History of the McLean County Medical Society* (1954), p. 179.

[24] Dr. W3MP, p. 5.

[25] ibid., p. 9.

[26] Dr. B2MP, p. 3.

[27] Dr. V1MP, p. 7.

[28] Dr. S1MP, pp. 8, 11.

[29] Dr. O1MP, p. 6.

[30] Dr. T2MP, p. 2.

[31] Livingston, op.cit., p. vii.

[32] Dr. W3MP, pp. 12-13.

[33] ibid., pp. 4-5.

[34] Dr. S1MP, p. 12.

[35] Dr. B2MP, pp. 2-3.

[36] Dr. O1MP, pp. 8-9.

[37] Dr. W3MP, pp. 15-17.

[38] Dr. S1MP, p. 11.

[39] ibid., p. 16.

[40] Dr. T2MP, p. 2.

[41] Dr. O1MP, p. 4.

[42] ibid.

[43] ibid., p. 8.

[44] ibid., p. 12.

[45] Dr. V1MP, pp. 4, 6.

[46] Dr. S1MP, p. 13.

[47] Dr. V1MP, pp. 10-11.

[48] Dr. S1MP, p. 19.

[49] ibid., pp. 21-22.

262

[50] Dr. S1MP, pp. 22-23.
[51] Dr. O1MP, pp. 7, 9.
[52] Dr. V1MP, p. 12.
[53] Dr. D1MP, pp. 9-10.
[54] Dr. V1MP, p. 14.
[55] Dr. W3MP, p. 21.
[56] Dr. S1MP, pp. 29-30.
[57] Dr. O1MP, pp. 12-13.
[58] Dr. V1MP, p. 20
[59] Dr. W3MP, pp. 41, 46, 47.
[60] Dr. B2MP, p. 2.
[61] Dr. O1MP, pp. 13-14.
[62] Dr. S1MP, pp. 55, 58.
[63] ibid., p. 57.
[64] Dr. V1MP, p. 16.
[65] Dr. T2MP, p. 8.
[66] Dr. V1MP, p. 33.
[67] Dr. D1MP, p. 17.
[68] Dr. S1MP, pp. 30-31.
[69] Dr. B1MP, pp. 4, 5.
[70] Dr. W3MP, p. 6.
[71] ibid., pp. 24-25.
[72] Dr. S1MP, p. 32.
[73] ibid., p. 33.
[74] ibid., pp. 36-37.
[75] Dr. W3MP, p. 30.
[76] Dr. S1MP, p. 35.
[77] ibid., p. 39.
[78] ibid., p. 40.
[79] Dr. B2MP, p. 6.
[80] Dr. T2MP, pp. 8, 9, 12.
[81] ibid., p. 14.
[82] Dr. B2MP, p. 5.
[83] Dr. T2MP, p. 13.
[84] ibid., p. 19.
[85] Dr. O1MP, p. 20.
[86] Dr. S1MP, pp. 62, 66.
[87] Dr. V1MP, pp. 34-36.
[88] Livingston, op.cit., pp. 2-3.
[89] ibid., p. 4.
[90] Dr. T2MP, pp. 31-32.
[91] ibid., pp. 19-20.
[92] Dr. B2MP, p. 11.
[93] Dr. O1MP, p. 42.
[94] Livingston, op.cit., p. 11.
[95] Dr. S1MP, p. 51.
[96] Dr. O1MP, pp. 23, 24.
[97] Dr. V1MP, p. 37.
[98] Dr. T2MP, p. 15.
[99] Dr. O1MP, p. 27.
[100] Dr. V1MP, p. 40.

101 Starr, *Social Transformation.*, p. 385.

102 Dr. T2MP, p. 32.

103 Dr. O1MP, p. 39.

104 Dr. T2MP, p. 22.

105 Dr. S1MP, p. 57.

106 Dr. O1MP, p. 37.

107 Dr. S1MP, pp. 61-62.

108 Dr. B2MP, p. 14.

109 Dr. O1MP, pp. 22-23.

110 Mrs. S2MP, pp. 53-54.

111 Livingston, op.cit., p. 19.

112 Dr. B2MP, p. 15.

8. In Living Memory: The Experience of Health, Illiness and Medical Care in McLean County

1 Twenty-nine interviews were conducted in 1994-5 by volunteers associated with the *A Matter of Life and Death: Health, Illness and Medicine in McLean County* project. With one or two exceptions, these interviews were based on three questionnaires (tailored, respectively, for nurses, medical practitioners and lay people) developed for this project. Three interviews were conducted by Cynthia Baer in 1993; these interviews were based upon a questionnaire similar to that developed for lay respondents and are used with Ms. Baer's permission. Eight interviews were conducted by members of the Bloomington-Normal Black History Project during the 1980s; these interviews are used with the permission of the Bloomington-Normal Black History Project.

2 Mrs. W1MP, p. 26.

3 Mrs. A1MP, p. 32.

4 Isaac D. Rawlings, *The Rise and Fall of Disease in Illinois*, Vol. 2, Springfield, IL: Schnepp & Barnes (1927; reprinted 1994), pp. 58, 61.

5 This project is indebted for this information to the file on polio assembled in 1994 by Preston Hawks of the McLean County Historical Society .

6 Rawlings, op.cit., pp. 58, 61.

7 Karen A. Walters, "McLean County and the Influenza Epidemic of 1918-1919," unpublished paper written for the History of Illinois class at Illinois State University in 1980.

8 This treatment, hailed by some medical historians as the first true "antibiotic," was neither a quick fix, nor was it entirely safe. According to one authority, "For all its great advance in the treatment of syphilis, Salvarsan was still not a very good drug, requiring many painful injections before a cure could be pronounced. It was not until the advent of penicillin that the spread of syphilis was slowed." (Jenny Sutcliffe and Nancy Duin, *A History of Medicine*, New York: Barnes and Noble (1992), p. 101. According to one oral history respondent for this project, in McLean County syphilis continued to be treated with mercury until penicillin became available. (Mrs. L1MP, p. 15).

9 *Home Care of Communicable Diseases*, Boston, MA: John Hancock Mutual Life Insurance Company (1942), p. 5.

10 Sutcliffe and Duin, op.cit., p. 155.

11 *Home Care*, op.cit., p. 4.

[12] ibid., pp. 13-14.

[13] Mrs. C1MP, p. 30

[14] Mr. W4MP, pp. 42-43.

[15] Mrs. A1MP, p. 20.

[16] Mrs. F1MP, pp. 26-27.

[17] Mrs. B1MP, p. 11.

[18] Mrs. F2MP, p. 9.

[19] Mrs. H2MP, p. 4.

[20] Mr. W4MP, p. 29.

[21] Sutcliffe and Duin, *History of Medicine*, p. 111.

[22] Mrs. F2MP, p. 19.

[23] Mrs. R1MP, p. 7. Mrs. Rittenhouse (Mrs. R1MP), Mrs. Rueger (Mrs. R2MP) and Mrs. Rohm (Mrs. R3MP) (not these respondents' real names) (Cynthia Baer transcripts).

[24] Mrs. W1MP, pp. 18-21.

[25] Dr. S1MP, p. 36.

[26] Mr. F2MP, p. 25.

[27] Oral history transcript included in Mildred Pratt (ed), *We the People Tell Our Story*, Bloomington-Normal Black History Project, Illinois State University (no date), p. 18.

[28] Mrs. C1MP, pp. 14-15.

[29] Pratt, op.cit., p16.

[30] Mrs. W1MP, pp. 12-13.

[31] Mrs. A1MP, p. 29.

[32] Mr. S3MP, p. 19.

[33] Mrs. W1MP, p. 12; Pratt, op.cit., p. 16.

[34] Mrs. C1MP, p. 23. See also Mrs. F1MP, p. 25.

[35] Pratt, op.cit., p. 16.

[36] Mrs. C1MP, p. 16.

[37] Mrs. F1MP, p. 20.

[38] Pratt, op.cit., p. 16.

[39] Mrs. W1MP, p. 13.

[40] Mrs. C1MP, p. 15. See also Pratt, op.cit., p. 16.

[41] Mrs. C1MP, p. 15.

[42] Mrs. C2MP, p. 20.

[43] Mrs. E1MP, pp. 41-2.

[44] Mrs. C1MP, p. 16.

[45] ibid., pp. 18, 19.

[46] Mrs. B1MP, p. 13.

[47] Mrs. W1MP, pp. 13-14.

[48] ibid., p. 28.

[49] Dr. B2MP, p. 13

[50] Mr. F2MP, p. 24.

[51] Mrs. A1MP, pp. 25-26.

[52] ibid., p. 28.

[53] Mr. F2MP, p

[54] *Biographical History of the McLean County Medical Society, 1854-1954*, McLean County Medical Society (1954), p. 66.

[55] Mr. F2MP, pp. 23, 24, 26.

[56] Mrs. C2MP, p. 19, 20.

[57] Mr. W4MP, pp. 22-23.

58 Mrs. F1MP, p. 23.
59 Mr. W4MP, p. 39.
60 Mrs. A1MP, p. 26.
61 Mr. S3MP, p. 19.
62 Mr. W4MP, p. 38.
63 ibid., p. 15.
64 ibid., pp. 35, 36, 37.
65 Dr. V1MP, p. 35.
66 Mrs. W1MP, p. 16.
67 Mrs. F1MP, p. 29.
68 Mr. F2MP, p. 26.
69 Mrs. F1MP, p. 13.
70 Mrs. E1MP, p. 23.
71 Mrs. R3MP, pp. 38-39.
72 Mrs. A1MP, p. 33.
73 "The Prophylactic Forceps Operation," *American Journal of Obstetrics and Gynecology* 1 (1920), p. 41, quoted in R. W. and D. C. Wertz, *Lying-In: A History of Childbirth in America*, New York: The Free Press (1977), p. 143.
74 Wertz, op.cit., pp. 150-6.
75 ibid., p. 165.
76 Mrs. S2MP, p. 3.
77 Mrs. R1MP, p. 6.
78 Mrs. R2MP, p. 7.
79 ibid., p. 21.
80 Mrs. A1MP, p. 32.
81 Mrs. C1MP, p. 20.
82 Bloomington-Normal Black History Project files.
83 ibid.
84 Mrs. C1MP, p. 20.
85 Mrs. B1MP, p. 19.
86 Mrs. C1MP, p. 22.
87 Mrs. A1MP, p. 33.
88 Mrs. R2MP, p. 21.
89 ibid., p. 20.
90 Mrs. W1MP, p. 30.
91 Mrs. E1MP, pp. 16-17.
92 Mrs. C1MP, p. 61.
93 Mr. S3MP, p. 23.
94 Mrs. E1MP, p. 16.
95 Mrs. R1MP, pp. 23-24.
96 Mrs. W2MP, p. 32.
97 Mrs. R3MP, p. 15.
98 Mr. W4MP, pp. 4-5.
99 *The Pantagraph*, 1/7/1996.
100 Bloomington-Normal Black History Project files. Lucinda Brent Posey interviews.
101 Mrs. W1MP, pp. 15-16.
102 ibid., Oscar Waddell interviews.
103 Bloomington-Normal Black History Project files. Lucinda Brent Posey interviews.

[104] Mr. W4MP, pp. 44-45.

[105] Mrs. W1MP, pp. 25-26.

[106] Bloomington-Normal Black History Project files. Lucinda Brent Posey interviews.

[107] See, e.g., Charles O. Jackson, "Death Shall Have No Dominion: The Passing of the World of the Dead in America," in Richard A. Kalish (ed.), *Death and Dying: Views From Many Cultures*, Farmington, NY: Baywood Publishing Co., (1980), p. 48; James J. Farrell, *Inventing the American Way of Death*, 1830-1920, Philadelphia, PA: Temple University Press (1980), pp. 146-8.

[108] Mrs. F1MP, pp. 35-36.

[109] See, e.g., Mrs. E1MP, Mr. W4MP, Mrs. A1MP, Mrs. F1MP.

[110] Mrs. B1MP, pp. 8-9.

[111] Mrs. A1MP, p. 36.

[112] ibid., p. 41.

[113] Mr. S3MP, p. 32.

[114] ibid., pp. 29-30.

[115] Mrs. B1MP, p. 9.

[116] Jessica Mitford, *The American Way of Death*, New York: Fawcett World Library, Crest Books (1963).

[117] Mrs. F1MP, p. 39.

[118] Mrs. A1MP, p. 46.

9. Conclusion: The Face in the Mirror

[1] These began with establishment of the ophthalmologists' board in 1916, which was followed by the otolaryngologists in 1924. The third examining board was founded by the obstetricians and gynecologists in 1930. Thereafter, specialty boards proliferated rapidly; by 1937, twelve had been established. "In 1940 the first edition of the Directory of Medical Specialists was published. For the first time, an elite within the profession received formal recognition." Paul Starr, *The Social Transformation of American Medicine*, New York: Basic Books (1982), pp. 356-7.

Bibliography

Primary Sources

"An Autobiography of Dr. Cyrenius Wakefield," revised by Dr. Homer Wakefield (1889?), unpublished ms., McLean County Historical Society

Biographical History of the Members of the McLean County Medical Society and Other Physicians Who Have Practiced Medicine in McLean County, 1854-1934, Bloomington, IL: McLean County Medical Society (1934)

Biographical History of the Members of the McLean County Medical Society, McLean County Medical Society (1954)

"Brokaw Hospital Annual Report" (1930), A. E. Livingston Health Science Library, BroMenn Healthcare, Bloomington, IL

DeLee, Joseph,"The Prophylactic Forceps Operation," American Journal of Obstetrics and Gynecology, 1 (1920)

Drake, Daniel, A Systematic Treatise Historical, Etiological, and Practical on the Principal Diseases of the Interior Valley of North America, Vol. 2, New York: Burt Franklin (1971 reprint: first published 1854)

Dickens, Charles, Martin Chuzzlewit, London (1843-4)

Essig, Maude, "History of Brokaw Hospital," unpublished ms., A. E. Livingston Health Science Library, BroMenn Healthcare, Bloomington, IL (1939)

Fishbein, Morris (ed.), Modern Home Medical Adviser, New York: Doubleday, Doran (1935)

Good Literature, New York: F.M. Lupton, January 1900

Home Care of Communicable Diseases, Boston, MA: John Hancock Mutual Life Insurance Company (1942)

The Home Cook Book of Chicago, Chicago, IL: J. Fred Waggoner (1874)

Kelso Sanitarium, Bloomingon, IL: Kelso Sanitarium (1916?)

Liquorian, vol. 57, no. 6 (1969)

The Pantagraph, Bloomington, IL (1879-1995)

The People's Home Journal, New York: F.M. Lupton (1900)

"Records of the McLean County Medical Society, 1891-1910," unpublished ms., McLean County Historical Society

Rogers, Thomas P., "Day Books, 1839-1854," McLean County Historical Society

"St. Joseph's Hospital Accounts, 1880-97," unpublished ms., The Sisters of the Third Order of St. Francis, Peoria, IL

"St. Joseph's Hospital Admissions Records, 1880-1906," unpublished ms., The Sisters of the Third Order of St. Francis, Peoria, IL

"St. Joseph's Medical Staff Records, 1885-1902," unpublished ms., The Sisters of the Third Order of St. Francis, Peoria, IL

Thackeray, William Makepeace, History of Pendennis, Vol. 2, London (1850)

The Wanamaker Diary, Philadelphia, New York and Paris (1910)

Weekly National Flag, Bloomington, IL (1856-9)

Transcripts of oral history interviews conducted for the "A Matter of Life and Death: Health, Illness and Medicine in McLean County" project are housed in the McLean County Historical Society, Bloomington, Illinois. Transcripts of interviews conducted for the Bloomington-Normal Black History Project are housed by that project at Illinois State University, Normal, Illinois.

Secondary Sources

Abel, Emily K., "Family Caregiving in the Nineteenth Century: Emily Hawley Gillespie and Sarah Gillespie, 1858-1888," Bulletin of the History of Medicine, vol. 68, no. 4, pp. 573-99.

Armstrong Beatrice, "Silas Hubbard, Early Physician of McLean County," unpublished ms., McLean County Historical Society

Avery, Kevin, "Privial Pursuit: A Research Paper on Outhouses," unpublished ms. (1985)

Barkan, Ilyse D., "Industry Invites Regulation: The Passage of the Pure Food and Drug Act of 1906," American Journal of Public Health, vol. 75, no. 1 (1985), pp. 18-26.

Bateman, Newton, (ed.), Historical Encyclopedia of Illinois and History of McLean County, Chicago, IL: Munsell Publishing Co. (1908)

Beecher, Catharine E., Letters to the People on Health and Happiness, New York: Arno Press and the New York Times (1972 reprint of the 1855 edition)

Beier, Lucinda McCray, Sufferers and Healers: The Experience of Illness in Seventeenth-Century England, London: Routledge and Kegan Paul (1987)

Bingham, A. Walker, The Snake-Oil Syndrome: Patent Medicine Advertising, Hanover, MA: The Christopher Publishing House (1994)

Blake, J. B., "From Buchan to Fishbein: The Literature of Domestic Medicine," in G. B. Risse, R. L. Numbers and J. Walzer Leavitt (eds), Medicine Without Doctors: Home Health Care in American History, New York: Science History Publications (1977), pp. 11-30.

Bonner, Thomas Neville, Medicine in Chicago, 1850-1950, Madison, WI: The American History Research Center (1957)

Boorde, Andrew, The Breviary of Health, London (1587)

Brieger, Gert H., "From Conservative to Radical Surgery in Late Nineteenth-Century America," in C. Lawrence (ed.), Medical Theory, Surgical Practice, London: Routledge and Kegan Paul (1992), pp. 216-31.

"BroMenn Healthcare Historical Program - Script" (1992)

Cassedy, James, Medicine in America: A Short History, Baltimore, MD: Johns Hopkins University Press (1991)

Cassedy, James, "Why Self Help? Americans Alone with their Diseases 1800-1850" in G. B. Risse, R. L. Numbers and J. Walzer Leavitt (eds), Medicine Without Doctors: Home Health Care in American History, New York: Science History Publications (1977), pp. 31-48.

<u>Danvers, Illinois Community History</u>, Danvers Historical Society, Inc. (1987)

Duis, Dr. E., <u>Good Old Times in McLean County</u>, Bloomington, IL: The Leader Publishing and Printing House (1874)

Esposito, Margaret, <u>Places of Pride: The Work and Photography of Clara R. Brian</u>, Bloomington, IL: McLean County Historical Society (1989)

Estes, Steven R., <u>Christian Concern for Health: The Sixtieth Anniversary History of the Mennonite Hospital Association</u>, Bloomington, IL: Mennonite Hospital Association (1979)

Farrell, James J., <u>Inventing the American Way of Death, 1830-1920</u>, Philadelphia, PA: Temple University Press (1980)

Ferguson Corlin, "The McLean County Poor Farm," unpublished report (1995)

Ferguson, Corlin, "Willow Bark Institute," unpublished report, McLean County Historical Society, Bloomington, IL (1995)

Fox, Daniel M., <u>Power and Illness: The Failure and Future of American Health Policy</u>, Berkeley, CA: University of California Press (1993)

Gegel, Brian T., "Formation and the First Fifty Years of the 6th District Illinois Nurses' Association," unpublished paper (1992), Illinois Wesleyan University

Gevitz, Norman, <u>The D.O.s: Osteopathic Medicine in America</u>, Baltimore, MD: Johns Hopkins University Press (1982)

Gevitz, Norman, <u>Other Healers: Unorthodox Medicine in America</u>, Baltimore, MD: Johns Hopkins University Press (1988)

Hasbrouck, Jacob, <u>History of McLean County Illinois</u>, Topeka-Indianapolis: Historical Publishing Company (1924)

<u>The History of McLean County, Illinois</u>, Chicago, IL: Wm. Le Baron, Jr., & Co. (1879)

Ingalls, Marlin Ray, "The Espy Pharmacy Records," unpublished Illinois State University Master's thesis (1986)

Jackson, Charles O., "Death Shall Have No Dominion: The

Passing of the World of the Dead in America," in Richard A. Kalish (ed.), <u>Death and Dying: Views From Many Cultures</u>, Farmington, NY: Baywood Publishing Co. (1980)

Kaufman, Martin, <u>Homeopathy in America: The Rise and Fall of a Medical Heresy</u>, Baltimore, MD: Johns Hopkins University Press (1971)

Latham, R., and W. Matthews (eds), <u>The Diary of Samuel Pepys</u>, vols. I-IX, Berkeley, CA: University of California Press (1970)

Leavitt, Judith Walzer, <u>Brought to Bed: Childbearing in America, 1750-1950</u>, Oxford University Press (1986)

Livingston, A. Edward, <u>A History of the Practice of Medicine in McLean County, Illinois 1930-1980</u>, privately published (1989)

Matejka, Michael, and Greg Koos, <u>Bloomington's C. & A. Shops: Our Lives Remembered</u>, Bloomington, IL: McLean County Historical Society (1987)

McNeill, William H., <u>Plagues and Peoples</u>, Garden City, NY: Anchor Press/Doubleday (1976)

<u>Mennonite Hospital School of Nursing: The Passing of the Flame</u>, Bloomington, IL: Mennonite College of Nursing (1985)

Morantz, Regiina, "The Lady and Her Physician," in Mary Hartman and Lois W. Banner (eds), <u>Clio's Consciousness Raised: New Perspectives on the History of Women</u>, New York: Harper & Row (1974), pp. 38-53.

Musser, Lori Ann, "Nursing Education at Illinois Wesleyan University: 1923 to 1976," unpublished paper (1976?), Illinois Wesleyan University

Orendorff, J. B., "Sketch of Omen and Zena Olney," unpublished ms., McLean County Historical Society

Orendorff, J.B., "Sketch of Major Baker," unpublished ms., McLean County Historical Society

Oyer, R. L., "Of Doctors and Sickness in Chenoa: A Historical Perspective," unpublished ms. prepared for the Chenoa Historical Society (1992)

Plummer, Linda K., "Medicine Factory," <u>Illinois History</u>, vol. 16, no.1 (1962), p. 10.

Pratt, Mildred (ed.), We the People Tell Our Story, Bloomington-Normal Black History Project, Illinois State University (no date)

Profile of Illinois' Elderly, Illinois Department on Aging (1994)

Rawlings, Isaac D., The Rise and Fall of Disease in Illinois, 2 vols., Springfield, IL: Schnepp & Barnes (1927; reprinted 1994)

Reverby, Susan M., Ordered to Care: The Dilemma of American Nursing, 1850-1945, Cambridge University Press (1987)

Risse, G. B., R. L. Numbers and J. Walzer Leavitt (eds), Medicine Without Doctors: Home Health Care in American History, New York: Science History Publications (1977)

Rosen, George, Preventive Medicine in the United States, 1900-1975, New York: Science History Publications (1975)

Rosenberg, Charles, The Care of Strangers: The Rise of America's Hospital System, New York: Basic Books (1987)

Charles Rosenberg, The Cholera Years, University of Chicago Press (1962)

Rothman, Sheila M., Living in the Shadow of Death: Tuberculosis and the Social Experience of Illness in American History, Baltimore, MD: Johns Hopkins University Press (1994)

Stage, Sarah, Female Complaints: Lydia Pinkham and the Business of Women's Medicine, New York: W. W. Norton & Co. (1979)

Starr, Paul, The Social Transformation of American Medicine, New York: Basic Books (1982)

Stevens, Rosemary, In Sickness and in Wealth: American Hospitals in the Twentieth Century, New York: Basic Books (1989)

Sutcliffe, Jenny and Nancy Duin, A History of Medicine, New York: Barnes and Noble (1992)

Tate, H. Clay, The Way it was in McLean County, 1972-1822, Bloomington, IL: McLean County History '72 Association (1972)

Walitschek, David A., "Historic Archaeological Investigations at the Reuben Benjamin House," unpublished Master's thesis, Illinois State University (1988)

Walters, Karen A., "McLean County and the Influenza Epidemic of 1918-1919," unpublished paper, Illinois State University (1980)

Wertz, R. W. and D. C., Lying-In: A History of Childbirth in America, New York: The Free Press (1977)

Young, James Harvey, The Medical Messiahs: A Social History of Health Quackery in Twentieth-Century America, Princeton University Press (1967)

Young, James Harvey, "Patent Medicines and the Self-Help Syndrome," in G. B. Risse, R. L. Numbers and J. Walzer Leavitt (eds), Medicine Without Doctors: Home Health Care in American History, New York: Science History Publications (1977), pp. 95-116.

Zeuch, Lucius, History of Medical Practice in Illinois, Vol. 1, Chicago: The Book Press (1927)

Index